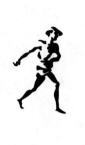

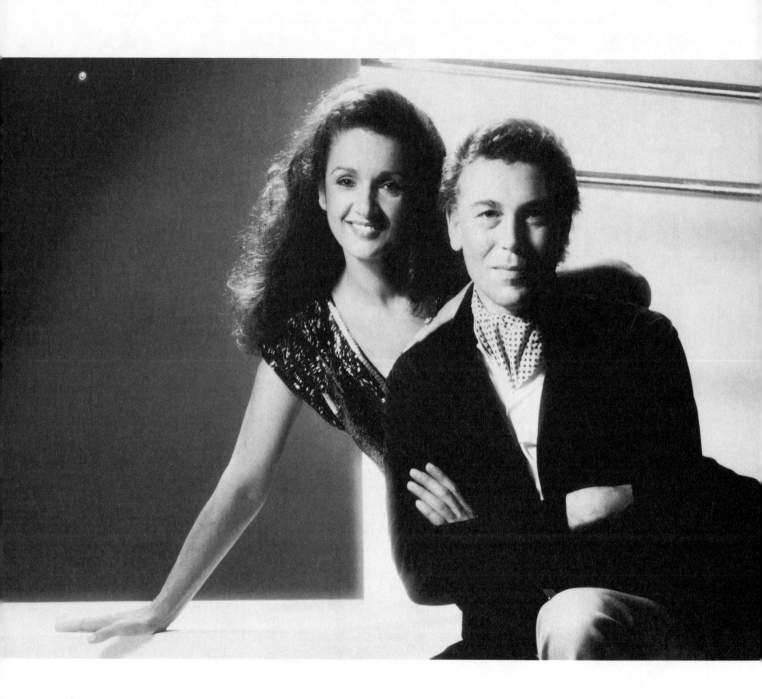

THE CHADWICK SYSTEM

Discovering the Perfect Hairstyle for _You_

JOHN AND SUZANNE CHADWICK

Illustrations by John Chadwick
Photographs by Roy Volkmann

SIMON AND SCHUSTER • NEW YORK

Published by Simon and Schuster
A Division of Gulf & Western Corporation
Simon & Schuster Building
Rockefeller Center
1230 Avenue of the Americas
New York, New York 10020
SIMON AND SCHUSTER and colophon are trademarks of Simon & Schuster
Designed by Eve Metz
Manufactured in the United States of America

10 9 8 7 6 5 4 3 2 1

Library of Congress Cataloging in Publication Data
Chadwick, John, date.
   The Chadwick system.

   1. Hairdressing. I. Chadwick, Suzanne.
II. Title.
TT972.C48   1982   646.7'242   82-10461

ISBN 0-671-44016-0

Frontispiece photograph by Roget Prigent

Acknowledgments

We would like to thank our parents and family for their encouragement. Also, Rhonda Racz, our "PR," who was the first to say "you've got to write a book," and insisted we did; Kathleen Beckett, our writer, whose patient unraveling of our thoughts produced the chapters; Wendy Lipkind, our agent, for her sensitive concern; Carmine Minardi and David Velasco, our creative directors, who worked on the concept, cutting guides, and illustration placement; and Anne Bartlett, our personal secretary, for hours spent "beyond the call of duty." In addition, we would like to thank:

Terry Foster and Danny Velasco, creative directors, for all the superb assistance with the many photo sessions, and for being there for ten years.

Roy Volkmann for photography; Ariella for makeup; Patty Wilson and Sarah Hilton for wardrobe.

To Pearl Octaviano, Larry Albus, Joanne Melende, Z of New York, thank you.

Special thanks to our lifelong friends and colleagues.

Gerald Duval for providing over the years all the many white elephants with pink spots at the drop of the hat.

Jamison Shaw, Charles Eichel, Fred Norton, Jim Metcalf, Irving Sherman, Edward Gadd, Harry Robbins, Joanna Brown, Art Shoffner, Seymour Finkelstein, Leonard Benson, Irene Frangides, Donn Byrne.

To Jack Shor, vice-president of public relations, Clairol, thank you for your quiet strength; Roger Tucker for the art direction; Phyllis Klein and Nancy Coleman for their advice. To all our friends and associates at Clairol, our special thanks for all their contributions and kindnesses . . . and especially to all our hairdressing friends for their love and support.

Dedicated with love
to our daughter, Rebecca.
"You bring the sunshine every day."

CONTENTS

Introduction   11

1. Texture   15

2. Formation   17

3. Quantity   19

4. Finding Your Hair Type   20

5. How to Change Your Hair . . .
   Straightening, Coloring, and
   Perming   23

6. Timing   31

7. Skill Rating   33

8. The Tools You Need   36

9. Your Hair, Your Face, and Your Body   47

10. The Haircut—Key to the Perfect
    Hairstyle   57

11. How to Find the Perfect Hairdresser   67

12. How to Talk to Your Hairdresser   71

13. The Best Products for Your Hair   74

14. Transition Hair: How to Grow Out
    What You Don't Like   78

15. Creating Your Own Home
    Hair-Grooming Center   81

16. Discovering the Perfect Hairstyle for
    You   86

The Chadwick Hairstyles   89

INTRODUCTION

What is the single biggest problem a woman has with her hair? *Finding a style she likes that is right for her*—which is to say right for her hair as well as for her face and features.

The Chadwick System is designed especially for you to take the guesswork, frustration, and disappointment out of this search— to help you find exactly what you want: a hairstyle that is perfect for you. In addition, the Chadwick System gives you complete, easy-to-follow directions on how to create your perfect hairstyle yourself.

FINDING YOUR PERFECT HAIRSTYLE

What do we mean by "perfect hairstyle"? It's a style that not only looks good on you, flattering your facial features and body proportions, but fits in comfortably with your life-style. Your perfect hairstyle takes only the amount of time you're willing to give; it requires a skill level to achieve and maintain that you already possess or can learn easily.

WHAT IS THE CHADWICK SYSTEM?

The Chadwick System is a totally *new* concept in hairstyling— and it works. The key to our system and to your success: It's *personal.* Everyone's hair differs and requires special, unique treatment. For example, if you have fine, straight, thin hair and someone else has coarse, curly, thick hair, you're both going to need a completely different set of instructions to achieve the same hairstyle. We give those personalized instructions in this book. And we guide you to the styles that do the most for your particular type of hair . . . styles that work with fine, straight, thin hair with the least amount of fuss and the best, longest-lasting results; styles that do the same for coarse, curly, thick hair; and styles that are best suited for the entire range of hair in between.

There's nothing general about the Chadwick System. We've broken down hair into *twenty-seven different types.* Once you establish which type you are, you'll find all the specific information you need to make the most of your hair.

WHAT YOU'LL FIND IN THIS BOOK

We've created and photographed forty great-looking hair-styles, with enough variety to satisfy any woman's particular taste. In charts that accompany each style, we tell you just what you, with your unique hair type, will have to do to get the style. We've taken away the guesswork. We're honest—we tell you right up front whether the style is a good bet for you to try. If it isn't, we give you advice on what you can do to your hair to make the style possible. If it is a good choice for you to try, we tell you how much time—for you personally—it will take to create the style . . . and how much skill you'll need. Right away you can see if the style is compatible with the time and skill you possess. We tell you exactly what hair-care equipment you will need and give special illustrated tips to show you how to use these tools to get the style you want. In addition, for each of the forty hairstyles described, you'll learn which facial features the style hides, which it highlights, and which body proportions it flatters. The result: Not only will your hair look better, you will, too!

Finally, for each style there is a detailed sketch with specific instructions regarding the key to any successful hairstyle: the cut. To get the cut you need for your hairstyle, all you have to do is show the appropriate sketch to your hairdresser.

With these easy-to-follow, step-by-step directions, you'll discover what thousands of professional hairdressers and happy women already know—the Chadwick System is *foolproof,* guaranteed to give you a perfect hairstyle. There's no way you can miss!

WHO WE ARE

We are professional hairdressers who *love* what we do and get our biggest satisfaction from helping women choose a hairstyle that makes them look absolutely great! We have spent twenty years developing this system . . . twenty years in which we've had more contact with more women and what they look for and want in hair care than any other hairdressers.

We started hairdressing in England (we both come from hairdressing families) and came to the United States in 1963 to introduce the blow-dry styling revolution to these shores. Since our arrival, we've trained hairdressers from all over the world for the two top international hair salon chains in leading department stores. We've trained approximately thirty thousand hairdressers, now working in the best salons in twenty-six countries—

from Harrods in London to Bergdorf Goodman in New York to Neiman-Marcus in Texas to Saks in California . . . to, we wouldn't be surprised, the hairdressers in your favorite department store. We travel around the world to keep abreast of the latest techniques, trends, and innovations in hairstyling and distill what we see to teach other professionals who want to stay current with the news in hair. They, in turn, keep us posted on what their clientele wants. And, as creative consultants for Clairol, we put this exchange of information to work, creating a yearly collection of hairstyles that go with the latest in fashion, forecasting trends for the coming year, giving styling and product direction, appearing on television and in special presentations around the country. We've been called "the hairdressers' hairdressers," and we want to put this professional knowledge, our teaching experience and trade secrets, to work for you!

YOU AND YOUR HAIR

What the system requires on your part: one simple thing, to understand your hair. As we said, the key to this system—what makes it foolproof—is that it's personal. It's going to tell you, individually, how to love and care for your hair so that it will look its best. So, first you need to know just what kind of hair you have—that is, you need to find your own unique *hair type*. That's all. Once you know your hair type, you'll understand what your hair will or will not do, and exactly how to make it do what you want it to.

Let's get started!

WHAT THE CHADWICK SYSTEM WILL SHOW YOU

- The hairstyles that are most compatible with your individual hair type
- How to recognize your individual hair type—texture, formation, and quantity
- How long it will take you to style your hairstyle choice
- The techniques and styling skills each individual hair type requires for each style
- The tools and appliances you'll need for each individual hairstyle and hair type
- Which facial features each style hides and highlights
- Which body proportions each hairstyle flatters
- If the hairstyle you choose is a Minimum Care style that requires the least amount of time for the longest-lasting results . . . or
- If the style is a Temporary style that lasts for a limited period of time
- Detailed illustrations for each hairstyle, including directions for cutting, layering, and shaping to take to your hairdresser

1 TEXTURE

The first thing you need to know to help you find your individual hair type is your hair's *texture*.

Hair texture can be *fine, medium,* or *coarse*—it all depends on the thickness of each hair strand. Texture is not the same thing as the quantity of your hair—the number of hairs you have on your head. Your hair's texture depends upon the fineness or thickness, called coarseness, of each hair's diameter, or denier. Here are some easy ways to help you determine what hair texture you have:

Fine texture—Hair is usually shiny, particularly if it is also straight, and as light and weightless as a feather, as soft as silk. It doesn't hold a curl. . . . If you set it and thirty minutes later the curl has drooped, that's a good signal your hair is fine. Or: Stand in front of a mirror holding your palms straight in front of and a few inches away from your face. Now blow. If your hair moves, it's probably fine. Another test: Spray your hair lightly with a mist bottle—if it dampens easily, chances are it's fine. If it "sinks" or clings to your head while you sleep, leaving you with "deflated" hair in the morning, it's probably fine. If it sinks to your head when the weather is humid, most likely it's fine. One more test: Gather up a large section of hair and push back the ends against your palm. If it feels like a baby's brush, you have fine-textured hair.

Coarse texture—Coarse hair has a thick denier and feels heavy. It is usually dull. If you gather up a large section of hair, push it back against your palm, and get the feel of a paint brush, your hair texture is coarse. If, after sleeping, or after being exposed to humidity, your hair strands seem to expand and get much fuller, that's another indication that it is coarse.

Medium texture—You fall into this category if at times your hair has all the qualities and passes all the tests of fine texture . . . and, at other times, as it responds to changes in the weather and changes in your body cycle, seems like coarse texture. Medium-texture hair may feel coarse one week and fine the next week.

CHANGING TEXTURE

Certain products and procedures can temporarily alter your hair's texture, giving fine hair a bit of a boost; coarse hair slightly more silkiness.

If your hair is fine—Permanent tints or coloring products containing peroxide, such as those used in highlighting, will expand hair strands, actually making them thicker. So will perming—in two ways. First, by fattening each hair strand chemically . . . and, second, if your hair is straight, by giving it some curve so it doesn't just lie there, but makes the strands bounce against each other, creating the illusion of thicker hair. A "hot" solution perm (one that relies on heat to help activate the chemical reaction that breaks down and reforms your hair) might be too gentle to do the "fattening" job—you'll end up with the same feather-light texture nature gave you. A "cold" perm may be a better choice to help expand and thicken hair. Because there are so many types of perms available, it's best to ask your hairdresser which one he or she recommends. Fine hair can also be fattened with hair sprays and setting lotions.

If your hair is coarse—Nothing you or anyone can do will actually slim down your hair strands, but there are certain products—conditioners, henna, or semipermanent hair colors—that coat each hair strand and make hair shinier, more controlled, and more like fine hair.

If you have medium hair—Try the most temporary hair texture changers: hair spray or setting lotion when it's feeling fine . . . conditioners when it's coarse.

Note: For more information on the pros and cons of coloring and perming, see Chapter 5.

2 FORMATION

The second thing you need to know to determine your hair type is your hair's *formation*.

Is your hair *straight, wavy,* or *curly?*

There are many gradations of formation . . . from the needle-straight hair of many Asians, to hair with a slight curve, to deep waves, all the way to the frizzy hair of most blacks. Sometimes hair formation can vary on the same head—you might have straight hair along the front hairline, for instance, and curly hair over the ears and on the nape. The formation that predominates is your general hair formation. Don't confuse formation with cowlicks—they are shaped by a twist in your hair's growth direction (the angle at which a hair comes out of a pore in the scalp) but have nothing to do with whether that hair coming out is straight, wavy, or curly.

To tell which formation you have, shampoo your hair and let it dry naturally. Then hold a small section against the following sketches (snip a few strands if you want, or remove some hairs from a brush, wet them, and let them dry on the page). Which sketch does it most nearly match?

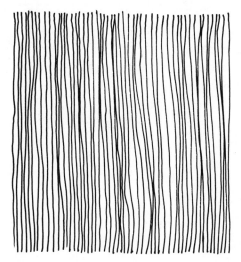

Straight

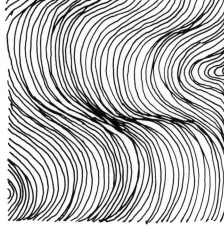

Wavy

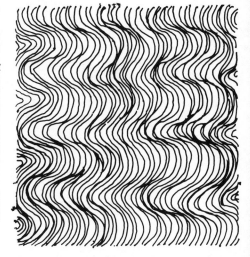

Curly

CHANGING FORMATION

If your hair is straight—The most obvious and lasting way to give it some curl or wave is with a permanent. Keep in mind, however, that if you get a nice, soft curl with a perm, it will probably last only twelve weeks, tops. If you decide to perm, ask your hairdresser which kind to have. . . . There are a wide variety available, and it takes a professional to weigh the pros and cons of each and then decide which is best for your particular type of hair. See Chapter 5 for a complete discussion of permanents. More temporary solutions to change straight hair: setting damp hair with pincurls or rollers, hot rollers, or a curling iron.

If your hair is wavy or curly—For a temporary change—lasting from a few minutes to a day or two, depending upon the weather and the individual—try straightening out hair with any of the following methods: a blow-dryer and brush, a curling iron used upside-down and pulled through the hair from the roots to the ends, a hot comb, a curling iron, hot rollers, a water-and-roller setting to make very curly hair into larger, looser curls, or plate irons. (**Note:** Plate irons should be used only by a professional who knows precisely how to control the heat.) You can also use straightening lotions—very carefully, especially if your hair is fine. As these lotions are quite potent, we do not recommend them for very long hair—they can make the hair "crack up" (see Chapter 5 for complete guidelines on straightening).

Another process we don't recommend: reverse perming, a method used to counteract the heaviness and deadness of frizzy hair that has been straightened and just lies there. In reverse perming, hair is permed on very large rollers to favor more curl than frizz, but the natural formation of the hair returns all too quickly, especially at the roots, which are very hard to reperm, and this consequently results in an unattractive growing-out period. It is far preferable for a woman with frizzy hair to become dextrous with temporary straightening changes. The best solution of all, however, is to get a good cut and find a style that works with—not against—your hair's natural formation. You'll find lots of beautiful possibilities in the hairstyle charts coming up.

3 QUANTITY

The third variable to help you find your personal hair type is *quantity*.

Quantity refers to the number of hairs per square inch on your head. Quantity can be *thin, medium, or thick* . . . and can vary on a single head. Many women have hair that is sparse around the temples, sides, and crown of the head and thicker around the ears and neckline. If the quantity of your hair varies, the type that predominates is your general hair quantity.

Some guidelines to help you determine what quantity you have:

Thin quantity—Make a ponytail. If it's as slim as a pencil, you probably have thin hair. Another good indication: If you can see your scalp when your hair is wet, it's probably thin. In general, blondes and redheads tend to have thinner hair quantity than brunettes, and finely textured hair tends to be thin in quantity.

Thick quantity—When you gather your hair into a ponytail, it looks like a horse's tail . . . You can't see the scalp when hair is wet, and, in general, you are a brunette and/or your hair is coarsely textured.

Medium quantity—Your ponytail is neither as thin as a pencil nor as thick as a horse's tail. Your scalp does not show through when your hair is wet, nor is it completely blanketed by hair.

Unfortunately, there is no reliable method to change the quantity of your hair—that is, to increase the number of hairs per square inch on your head. And, short of plucking out hairs, there's no way to decrease the quantity either. (You might get the illusion of less quantity with "effect cutting," in which a specialist cutter "adjusts" the midlength and end thickness of your hair—it takes a qualified eye and the skilled hands of a professional.)

4

FINDING YOUR HAIR TYPE

If you've read the preceding chapters on texture, formation, and quantity, you're now ready to go to the heart of the Chadwick System: finding your own individual *hair type*. Your *hair type is simply the combination of your hair's texture, formation, and quantity*—your TFQ Quotient—and knowing it is the key to finding the hairstyle that's perfect for you.

Look at the chart reproduced here. You'll see that there are twenty-seven different hair types. To see which one you are, write down the kind of texture, formation, and quantity hair you have. Now look at the chart and find the number that corresponds to the combination of your hair's characteristics. This number is your individual hair type.

For example, do you have fine-texture, wavy, medium-quantity hair? Then your hair type is number 5. If your hair is medium texture, straight, and thin, your hair type is number 10. If it is coarse texture, curly, and thick, your type is number 27, and so on.

Read the comments bracketed to the left of your hair type. These describe your individual hair type. They tell you your hair's characteristics, the hairstyles to which your hair is naturally suited, and what you can do to modify your hair so that it will be amenable to a greater number of styling options. For example, let's say your hair type is number 14—medium texture, wavy, and of medium thickness. This particular hair type has the most options for styling and is naturally suited to almost any hairstyle. Its stylability can, however, be improved upon by using color or having a curly perm (for more about changing your hair's natural characteristics, see Chapter 5).

TWENTY-SEVEN HAIR TYPES

hair tends to be limp, doesn't hold curl or wave;
hair is naturally suited to straight styles;
color adds body and control;
wavy perms only

hair tends to be delicate;
hair is naturally suited to wavy or curly looks;
color adds body and control;
straightening can damage

hair tends to be very delicate;
hair is naturally suited to curly styles;
color adds body and control;
straightening will damage

hair is easily styled, holds curl well;
hair is naturally suited to straighter styles;
color makes the set hold better;
wavy or curly perms

hair has most options for styling;
hair is naturally suited to almost any style;
color makes temporary straightening or curling
  hold better;
curly perms only

hair is easily styled;
hair is naturally suited to wavy or curly styles;
straightening will remove curl

hair tends to be porous and will overcurl;
hair is naturally suited to straighter, carefully cut
  styles;
subtle color helps the set hold better;
wavy perms only

hair tends to retain wave firmly;
hair is naturally suited to wavy or curly styles;
color makes temporary straightening or curling
  hold better

hair tends to be strong and obstinate;
hair is naturally suited to curly styles;
temporary color helps refine texture;
straightening will remove curl

TEXTURE	FORMATION	QUANTITY	HAIR TYPE
FINE	STRAIGHT	THIN	1
		MEDIUM	2
		THICK	3
	WAVY	THIN	4
		MEDIUM	5
		THICK	6
	CURLY	THIN	7
		MEDIUM	8
		THICK	9
MEDIUM	STRAIGHT	THIN	10
		MEDIUM	11
		THICK	12
	WAVY	THIN	13
		MEDIUM	14
		THICK	15
	CURLY	THIN	16
		MEDIUM	17
		THICK	18
COARSE	STRAIGHT	THIN	19
		MEDIUM	20
		THICK	21
	WAVY	THIN	22
		MEDIUM	23
		THICK	24
	CURLY	THIN	25
		MEDIUM	26
		THICK	27

As you look at the chart to find your individual hair type, keep in mind that certain combinations of hair characteristics give you more styling options than others. As a rule, *hair types that fall in the middle of the range of possible combinations have the greatest number of options for styling; hair types that fall at the outer or extreme ends of the range have the fewest number of styling options.*

If your hair type does not fall in the center of the range, or if you happen to like a hairstyle from one of the hairstyle charts in this book to which your hair is not naturally suited, don't despair. There *are* ways to alter or modify your hair that allow you to increase dramatically the number of your styling options. In the following chapter, we'll discuss the three most effective ways of doing this.

5
HOW TO CHANGE YOUR HAIR . . .
STRAIGHTENING, COLORING, AND PERMING

IMPROVING ON MOTHER NATURE

As we said earlier, certain of your hair's characteristics can be modified or altered to improve stylability and certain cannot. The *quantity* of your hair cannot be changed; however, the *texture* and *formation* of your hair can be altered.

The three most effective ways to alter your hair's texture and formation are by *straightening, coloring,* and *perming*. You can straighten hair or have a permanent to change the formation; color hair to change the texture. If you have an "extreme" hair condition—hair that's simply too fine or too curly to work with—one of these processes may be just the miracle lift you need to bring your hair closer to the desirable midrange of hair types and give you more styling options and flexibility than you ever thought possible.

SHOULD YOU CHANGE YOUR HAIR?

Our belief is that in general it is preferable to work with your hair's natural characteristics—its natural texture and formation. Why? Quite simply because keeping your hair the way it is naturally is *easier* than changing it. It requires less upkeep, and, in the long run, may wind up healthier than hair that has been altered continually. As a rule, women who keep their hair's natural tendencies find that the only real maintenance required is occasional cutting or trimming.

Many women, however, decide for very valid reasons that they want to change their hair's texture or formation. Usually this is because a woman is bored with her hair and the "look" she's had for a number of years or because she's found a style that is more becoming but requires some modification of her hair. The desire to change your hair's natural characteristics is quite common today, largely due to the high level of sophistication of coloring, straightening, and perming techniques now available. Just five years ago, when a woman got a wavy or curly perm, she took a chance that her hair would come out frizzy. Today, however, the chances of a perm giving you exactly the result you want are excellent. Changing or modifying your hair is easier, safer, and more reliable than ever before. If you do decide you want to change your hair's texture or formation, just be sure that you're willing to invest the extra time and money such changes require. This special investment will more than pay off in the way you feel about your hair.

Each of the following ways to alter your hair's characteristics has its own pros and cons, so read each one carefully before deciding which option(s) may be the answer for you. Then read the Special Hair-Care Regime we've included that tells you exactly what you need to do to maintain hair that's been straightened, colored, or permed.

STRAIGHTENING

Straightening can be very tricky. It makes hair more porous and can be damaging—especially to long hair—leaving you with broken, split ends if the hair is not carefully tended. It makes curly or wavy hair heavy, droopy, and needle straight. Moreover, it requires a high level of dexterity to put body or wave back into hair that's been straightened. And even if you succeed in doing this, the effect is only temporary. Women with very curly or frizzy hair, on the other hand, may find straightening worth the risks.

Our advice: If your hair type is number 1 to 8 on the chart, don't do it; number 9—it's still a risk, but if you want it done, go to an expert; hair types 13 to 18 and 22 to 27—you might try it, but you must have the dexterity, time, and products to take care of your hair once it's been straightened.

Straightened hair works best on *mid-length* hairstyles. Consider your body proportions and the facial features you want to hide or highlight (more about this in Chapter 9). If long hair is a more flattering choice for you, you should not straighten your hair.

HAIR QUALITY—WHAT IT IS, WHAT IT MEANS

The quality of your hair is based on its *porosity*, which is determined by the cortex–cuticle ratio of your hair strands. The cortex is the hair's fibrous central core; the cuticle is the hard, shiny outer layer. Fine-textured hair is 60 percent cortex and 40 percent cuticle. Medium hair is 75 percent cortex and 25 percent cuticle. Coarse hair is 90 percent cortex and 10 percent cuticle.

Too much cuticle can account for hair's glassiness and inability to hold a set; too little cuticle results in hair that looks and acts like a Brillo pad.

On some of the hairstyle charts, you'll find a note to add 25 percent extra preparation time for very porous hair—hair that is not good quality and requires more time to dry.

How do you know if your hair is very porous? It is if it

● wets down quickly with a mist bottle or "collapses" when it rains

● has the consistency of cooked spaghetti when wet—if you pull it, it will stretch and break easily

● looks burned and brittle when dry

● does not shine

● has split, dull, damaged ends

These conditions are usually caused by chemical or mechanical abuse . . . by using products or equipment improperly. Your hair is in the bad-quality category if it has been overpermed, overcolored, overstraightened, or damaged by improper brushing, combing, or drying. See the Special Hair-Care Regime at the end of this chapter for how to coax bad-quality hair into better shape.

COLORING

Hair coloring is more than just a way to cover gray. It's a hair cosmetic, capable of flattering skin tones, facial features, hairstyles—enhancing your entire appearance, brightening your whole outlook. Equally important is the stylability color can provide; those of you with hair types 1 to 18 on the chart are in for a pleasant surprise. Coloring can "boost" your texture, fattening fine, feathery hair, increasing its manageability and style options. This type of hair, however, is the kind that also has to be most careful of color; it's susceptible to overcoloring and abuse, so be careful—and subtle—and follow the Special Hair-Care Regime at the end of this chapter religiously. If you have coarse hair, types 19 to 27 on the chart, color will work best for you if you stick to slight color changes—a few shades lighter or darker overall, or techniques like highlighting, which affect only selected strands of hair. Again, be sure to follow the Special Hair-Care Regime conscientiously.

You'll often hear that it's best to go to a hairdresser for coloring, and it is, especially for the special treatments described later. However, the fact is that slight-change color can be done at home and look absolutely great. Be sure to read the instructions carefully and know if you are using a rinse that washes away after each shampoo, color that lasts through four to six shampoos, or a permanent color-change product (anything that lightens hair is permanent).

If you use henna, be aware that too-frequent applications can build up and give you a permanent color change. Full-head color change requires constant touching up as regrowth roots start to show. Highlighting, frosting, tipping, or some of the techniques you'll find described below don't show roots as obviously and don't require frequent touch-ups. Remember, the more you color, the more closely you must follow the Special Hair-Care Regime at the end of this chapter. If you are doing your own color, stick with the tried-and-true products. Seventy-five percent of all professional salons in the United States use coloring products made by Clairol, and for a good reason—they work and are compatible with other chemical changes you may do to your hair (straightening or perming, for instance). Don't experiment with new, never-seen-before products, and steer clear of those containing metallic dyes—they are not always compatible with other products. Talk to your hairdresser and consider naturalizing, selective shading, or the other processes described here. They're the best way to "fool" nature and improve your hair's characteristics with the least amount of fuss.

Hair-Coloring Terms

Rinse—Temporary hair color that lasts until you wash it out.

Semipermanent—Color that lasts through four to six shampoos. Cannot lighten hair. Comes in foam or lotion formulas.

Permanent—Does not wash out. Can lighten as well as darken hair. There are four main types of permanent hair color:

Shampoo-in tint—produces a color based on your natural shade in combination with the shade of hair coloring used. Can lighten hair a few shades or intensify or darken your natural color. Works in approximately twenty minutes.

Creme formula—Usually used for hair with gray or white that is resistant to color change, for long hair, and for maximum lightening with a one-step hair coloring. It is applied first to the new growth only and later brought down over the ends of the hair. Developing time is up to forty-five minutes.

Two-step blonding—Produces pale blond on hair that is fairly dark or has red undertones. First step removes pigment from your hair with lightener. Second step adds the shade of blond you want with toner.

Special effects—Any of dozens of techniques that accent your hair in a designated area. These include:

Highlighting, streaking, frosting—Use of a tint or mild bleach to change or lighten the color of selected strands of hair.

Lowlighting—Use of a tint to darken the color of selected strands of hair.

Naturalizing, or *selective shading*—Tone-on-tone effect for any hair color.

Sunshining—Soft blend of selected strands of blond or brown hair, which are lightened and toned.

Tortoise-shelling—Tone-on-tone effect for medium-to-dark brown hair, creating a warm, golden-brown shading.

Shading—Lightening hair around the face so that it gradually grows darker toward the back of the head.

Collaging—Multidimensional look using two lighter shades on short, curly hair.

Marbelizing—Light-and-dark tone-on-tone effect throughout the hair.

Dimensional hair coloring—Using two or three colors, usually similar in tone to the natural color, to give hair depth and contrast.

Tipping—Lightening tiny strands of hair in front.

Strand test—Preliminary test on a small section of hair before coloring or lightening entire head to see if the hair-coloring product will produce the result desired and to determine the mixture and developing time required.

Retouching—Coloring the new growth.

Stripping—Removal of virtually all color from the hair prior to applying another coloring.

PERMANENTS

Perming your hair will change its formation . . . and give you many more styling options. With perming, hair types 1 to 3 can acquire the characteristics of types 4 to 9; hair types 10 to 12 can become 14 to 18; and types 19 to 21 can become types 22 to 27. Permanents are wonderful for giving your hair the lift it needs. But before you try one, you should be aware that a perm is *not* for you if

- you have any bumps, scratches, or abrasions on your scalp
- you have bleached, double-process colored, or heavily frosted hair
- you have a record of allergic reactions to perm solutions

The key to getting a good perm doesn't lie in the bottle—it's determined by the length of your hair, the cut, the rod size, the processing time, and your hair's characteristics. A professional hairdresser can give you the best results with a perm. He or she will understand your hair's characteristics and know which kind of perm is best for you . . . as well as the safest, most efficient way to apply it.

In the hairstyle charts, we refer to two basic types of perms:

1. *Wavy* perms, which use medium-to-large rods to give you nice, soft waves. These perms usually last from six to twelve weeks. After the perm, your hair should match the sketch for *wavy* hair on page 17.
2. *Curly* perms, which use small-to-medium rods to give you lots of curl. This is a tighter perm than a wavy perm, and it lasts about eight to twelve weeks. Women with long fine hair should think twice before getting this kind of perm, as it may make your hair frizzy; similarly, a curly perm might make coarse-textured hair matted and hard to manage. After the perm, your hair should match the sketch for *curly* hair on page 17.

There is a third kind of perm, called a *body* perm. This type of perm leaves no discernible waves, but adds just enough body to give your hair a lift. Body waves generally last from four to six weeks.

Before giving you a perm, your hairdresser will make a test curl to give you an idea of how the perm will look and how it will affect your hair's condition. Trust the results of this test. And be sure to tell your hairdresser if you have had another perm or any coloring done on your hair within the last year—residues of these processes could still be lurking within your hair, especially at the ends.

Once you have your perm take proper care of it to help it last and look its best:

- Mist it into shape and style it with your fingers. Don't brush it— if hair is dry, brushing will make it woolly; if wet, it will eventually weaken the curl.
- Realize that if you blow-dry your hair straight or use rollers, hot rollers, or a curling iron, you are stretching out the curl and making the perm weaker. Brushing, shampooing—anything that pulls on the curl—is going to work out the perm, too.
- Realize, too, that if you ask for a soft perm it will not last as long as a tighter one, no matter how much extra money you may have paid for special attention or special lotions.
- Last, follow the Special Hair-Care Regime, described below, particularly if your hair is long or your natural hair type is number 1 to 9.

SPECIAL HAIR-CARE REGIME

If your hair has been straightened, colored, or permed . . . if it's long . . . if it's fine textured . . . if it's in bad shape—follow these steps to put it back in good condition:

- Have ends trimmed often.
- Shampoo carefully. Condition often using creme rinse to detangle coarse textures followed by a "coating" conditioner; leave on protein conditioners for fine textures. (See Chapter 13 for more on selecting the right conditioner.)
- Use your fingers and the force of the shower spray during your final rinse to help work out tangles.
- To dry hair, squeeze out excess water and pat—don't scrub— with a towel.

- "Natural" air drying is best. Just as too much sun can damage skin, too much heat can damage hair. Used in moderation, however, heat drying can help give a lift to your hair. A good technique is to wait until your hair is nearly dried by the air before applying heat. Also, when using a dryer, try one of the products specially made to help protect hair from the heat of drying.
- Use your fingers or a wide-tooth comb to style hair.
- If you must brush hair, don't do it frequently or vigorously (see Chapter 8 to find out which type of brush is best for you).
- When styling hair, don't twist it up tightly or screw in rollers snugly. Use wide cotton thread rather than covered bands to secure hair when making braids or rolls—just twist thread around ends and knot. To remove, cut thread carefully.
- To reduce static, wash brushes and combs in an antistatic detergent—the same as you would use for your laundry—or wipe hair with a sheet of antistatic product.
- If your hair's condition is too far gone for the techniques in this regime to be effective, your best alternative is to cut it and treat it better in the future!

6 TIMING

For each of the forty hairstyles included for you to select from in the charts that follow, we've indicated a start-to-finish time under the heading "Timing." *Timing* tells you how long it will take you to go from a wet head of shampooed hair all the way to the final photographed style—that is, the time it takes to dry and set or style your hair. Timing varies from as little as five minutes to as much as forty-five minutes, depending upon the complexity of the style you choose and the length, texture, and formation of your hair. For many of the hairstyles, the timing is enhanced considerably, as these need only the simplest touch-ups to be revived and to look great for one or two more days and nights.

When you look at the charts you will see that to get your perfect hairstyle, it's not always necessary to start out with a wet head of just-shampooed hair. If you have coarse or flyaway hair, for example, you might find that it's much more manageable to style the day *after* you have washed it. We've indicated on the charts those styles where this applies.

We also tell you on the charts whether the style is "Minimum Care" or "Temporary." Minimum Care styles work with your hair, stand up to the elements and the way you live, and require the least amount of effort. Temporary styles are great to try if you like to experiment with and vary your look . . . but expect to spend more time and attention on their upkeep. If you like the look and have the time and skill, they may be perfect for you. It's your choice!

HOW MUCH TIME SHOULD YOU SPEND?

The amount of time you need to achieve the hairstyle you want and to maintain it should be a consideration for you in deciding which hairstyles to try. Be honest about how much time you can really allocate to your hair. If mornings are a rushed, last-minute jumble for you, chances are a hairstyle that requires a thirty-five-minute start-to-finish time won't be compatible with your lifestyle. Keep in mind, though, that while some hairstyles require a relatively long start-to-finish time, they need very little touching up the next day to look as good as new. Other styles may require very little start-to-finish time but constant touchups (for example, misting the hair with water, using hot rollers or a curling iron, or just giving the hair a good brushing) during the day to stay in tiptop shape.

Keep in mind, too, that the more you fight nature—that is, changing the natural formation of your hair from, say, straight to curly—the more time you'll need. And, the longer, coarser, or thicker your hair is, the more time you'll need.

The best way to cut down on the time required to achieve the hairstyle or styles you want is to become more dextrous with your hair. If, for example, you know how to braid or roll your hair or control it with ornaments, you'll be able to vary your hairstyle in a minimum of time for a wonderful variety of looks. And the more dextrous you are, the less time it will take you to create and maintain any hairstyle you want. Take the quiz in the next chapter to find out your level of dexterity—your "skill rating."

7 SKILL RATING

The skill rating you need to achieve each of the forty hairstyles in this book is included on the hairstyling charts. Skill rating means your dexterity with brushes, combs, blow-dryers, and styling techniques—all the equipment, appliances, and procedures you use on your hair. Each style has a 1-to-5 skill rating number, which tells you at a glance just how much dexterity is required to achieve and maintain the style.

A skill rating of 1 means the style is very simple; 2—simple; 3—average; 4—moderately difficult; 5—difficult. To find your skill rating, take the following quiz:

QUIZ

1. Can you always make your hair look presentable? If *yes,* score 10 points; *sometimes*—5 points; *never*—0 points.

2. Can you part your hair from the front hairline to the nape in a continuous, straight, clean parting? If *yes,* score 10 points. If *no,* 0 points.

3. Can you neatly wind a hot roller in your hair? If *yes,* score 10 points. If *no,* score 5 points.

4. Can you neatly set all your hair on hot rollers? If *yes,* score 10 points. If *no,* score 5 points.

5. Can you make a curl with a curling iron? If *yes,* score 10 points. If *no,* score 0 points.

6. Can you bend your hair with a curling iron? If *yes,* score 10 points. If *no,* score 0 points.

7. Can you easily make a pincurl on the side of your head and secure it with a clip? If *yes,* score 10 points. If *no,* score 5 points.

8. Can you blow-dry your hair into a straight style with a brush and dryer? If *yes,* and you have curly hair, score 20 points. If *yes,* and you have wavy hair, score 10 points. If *yes,* and you have straight hair, score 5 points.

9. Can you bend or curve your hair into style with a brush and dryer? If *yes,* and you have curly hair, score 20 points. If *yes,* and you have wavy hair, score 10 points. If *yes,* and you have straight hair, score 10 points.

10. If you have long hair . . . can you gather it into a chignon? If *yes,* score 10 points. If *no,* 0 points.

11. If you have short hair, are you able to style it into another style variation? If *yes,* score 10 points. If *no,* score 0 points.

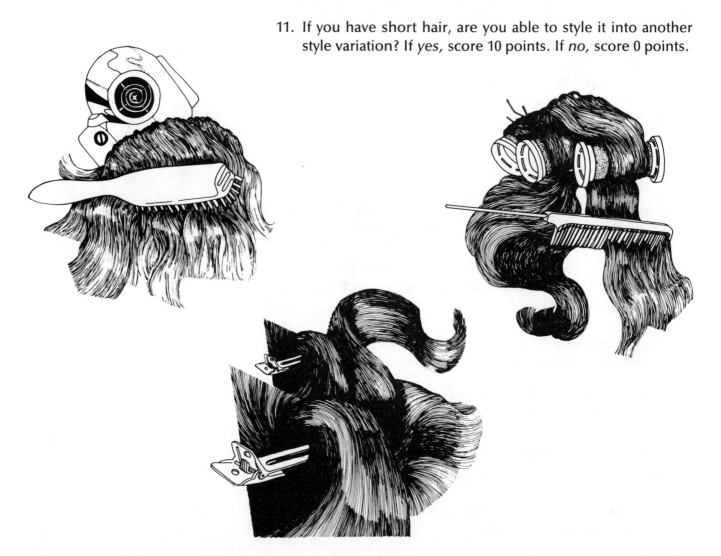

SCORING

Tally up the points to see how skillful you are:

- **0 to 20 points**
Attempt styles with a 1 or 2 skill rating.

  If you plan to try a hairstyle where it's necessary to change the natural formation or texture of your hair, your skill rating will need a lot of improvement. Your best bet is to find a hairstyle that works with your hair's natural tendencies.

- **21 to 40 points**
Attempt styles with a 1, 2, or 3 skill rating.

  You're pretty adept, but you're not a hairstyling whiz kid yet. With a little practice your choice of hairstyles can be greatly expanded.

- **41 to 60 points**
Attempt styles with a 1, 2, 3, or 4 skill rating.

  You've got a normal level of dexterity. Be sure to follow carefully the special tips on the chart of the hairstyle you select.

- **61 to 80 points**
Attempt styles with a 1, 2, 3, 4, and possibly 5 skill rating.

  You have a higher-than-average level of dexterity and can successfully create most hairstyles, including those where your hair's texture and formation must be altered.

- **81 to 100 or more points**
Anything goes! Styles with a 1, 2, 3, 4, or 5 skill rating are in your range.

  You are a hairstyling pro, and have the skill to achieve any style.

8 THE TOOLS YOU NEED

In the charts, under the heading "Tools and Appliances Required," you'll find a list of the various hair-care tools and equipment needed for setting, shaping, and styling the hairstyle. In this chapter, you'll find a description of these tools, plus a personal guide that tells you which ones you need for your specific hair type and which you need if you want to change your natural hair type to create a special hairstyle.

HAIRSTYLING'S BEST FRIEND: YOUR FINGERS

Before we discuss the various kinds of hair-care equipment used for styling, we want to introduce you to the "tool" that may be the single most valuable, and yet overlooked, of all: your fingers. Your fingers can *detangle* just-shampooed hair by working their way from the ends of your hair to your scalp (this is especially effective when you're standing under a shower as the force of the water stream aids detangling), *style* hair by pushing out and smoothing wavy and curly hair as you dry it, and *add shape and volume* to your hair. Watch how your hairdresser uses his or her fingers when styling your hair to learn how you can most effectively use this "tool."

WHAT TO LOOK FOR IN HAIR-CARE EQUIPMENT

To get the equipment you need to create the hairstyle you want at the best price requires some shopping around. Check out drug and department stores, discount centers, your own hair salon, and professional beauty supply shops (some sell to the public).

Now—the specifics. Here is an itemized guide to getting the best hair-care equipment available and using it properly for the best results.

Combs

Combs are available in a multitude of materials. Those of natural composition—wood, bone, horn—are usually expensive and easy to break or warp. Some people think that natural-composition combs are gentler on the hair than other combs, but in our view a tangle wrenched out with a natural-composition comb is just as damaging to the hair as one wrenched out with any other substance. Nor do we believe that natural-composition combs control static on dry hair. The best combs are made of *vulcanite, hard rubber,* or *smooth plastic*—they will stand up to cleansing with hot water and sterilizing liquid and to being dropped on the bathroom floor. Make sure a comb has no sharp edges or teeth. To check the quality of a comb, run a coin along the tips of the teeth to see if any are chipped, split, or snagged. If they are—get a new comb.

The following are various types of combs you might need:

- *Wide-tooth comb*—For detangling hair and combing conditioner through it with the least amount of damage.

- *Rattail comb*—For precision parting and setting, arranging and lifting a hairstyle. Watch out for ones with points that are too sharp.

- *Regular cutting comb*—A combination of wide and fine teeth. The best all-around comb. Use the wide end for getting out tangles, the fine end for parting or smoothing hair.

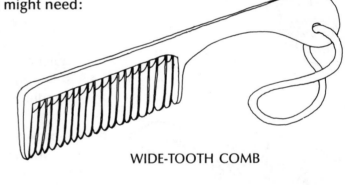

WIDE-TOOTH COMB

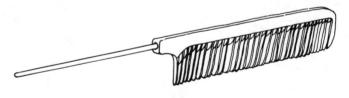

RATTAIL COMB

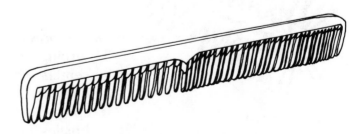

REGULAR CUTTING COMB

You should avoid

- *Short combs*—Handy for a back pocket or handbag, but not for any serious hairdressing where length in a comb is needed for manipulation.
- *Combination comb/brush*—Neither combs nor brushes well and is awkward to use.
- *Metal combs*—Indestructible to use—but very destructive to hair.

Brushes—Check the tips on your brush regularly to make sure they are in good condition and not damaging your hair. Never use a brush on wet hair until you have already used a wide-tooth comb to get all the tangles out.

The following are brushes you might need:

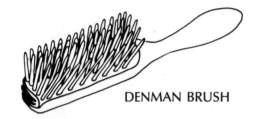

DENMAN BRUSH

- *Denman, or quill, brush*—The brush used most by professionals—rows of solid plastic teeth (quills) on a rubber base. This is the best all-purpose brush for stylng hair as well as drying it. (This brush does not hold moisture as bristle brushes do, which makes styling and drying proceed more quickly.) It comes in various sizes—we recommend the seven-row size for general use, the five-row size for your handbag.

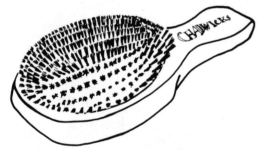

FLAT-BACK BRUSH

- *Flat-back bristle brush*—Usually a mixture of synthetic and natural bristles (100 percent natural bristles, unless they are the coarsest boar bristle, will not penetrate to the scalp) used for controlling (and reducing) the hair's volume. This brush adds shine and luster by spreading the hair's natural oils from the scalp to the tips.

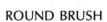

ROUND BRUSH

- *Round brush*—Used for ornamental effects: flipping bangs, turning under ends, forming curves. Some have metal centers, which, when used in conjunction with the heat of a blow-dryer, will make a curl quickly. Some have nylon spikes (better for fragile or fine hair) . . . others have bristles (better on coarse hair, but will tear fragile hair that tangles easily).

- *Vent brush*—This has short spikes set into a flat base with open vents to speed up drying time when using a blow-dryer. Also used to produce ridges in a hairstyle or enhance a precision cut—however, this is merely a temporary effect.

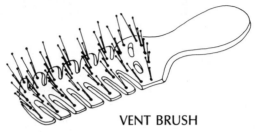

VENT BRUSH

Picks

Picks have wide-spaced prongs to lift curly hair and give it more volume and to separate hairs without causing frizziness.

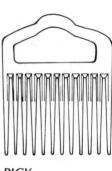

PICK

Blow-dryers

The market is flooded with blow-dryers, so it is very important that you know what to look for. Most professionals use 1500-watt dryers; as a rule, you should never go below 1000 watts, or you are only prolonging drying time. The blow-dryer you use should have easy-to-operate settings that let you regulate the amount of heat and air velocity. These settings should not be situated on the handle, where they might click off accidentally during use. There should be a protective grid or panel over the fan and a strong cord connection (you will be twisting it a lot). Attachments are usually unnecessary, except, if you have curly hair, you may want to use a diffuser.

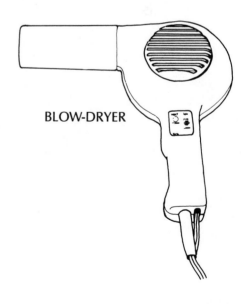

BLOW-DRYER

How to use—Bend head forward and begin drying hair at the back of the neck with the blow-dryer set at full power. Keep the nozzle four to five inches away from your head and move it around slightly while you dry your hair so that the air current is evenly distributed over the back of your head. When hair dries to the point where it is only slightly damp, return head to upright position, adjust dryer to half power and dry rest of head, again keeping the nozzle four to five inches away and moving it at all times. When hair is almost dry, begin any styling effects, such as turning hair up or under at the ends. When you've finished styling, your hair will be completely dry.

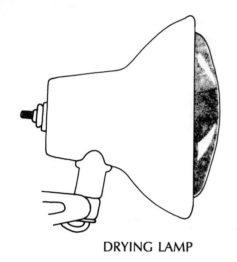

DRYING LAMP

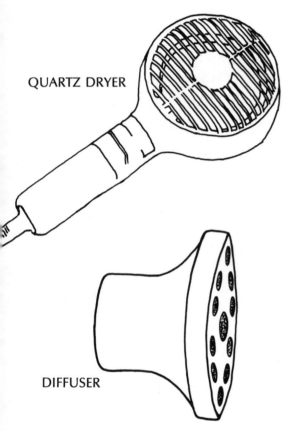

QUARTZ DRYER

DIFFUSER

Heat drying

If you have curly or wavy hair—natural or permed—heat hair drying may be best as it does not change the formation of the hair.

- *Heat lamps*—You will need at least two: one to dry the back of the head, one to dry the front. They are hard to position and may not be your most convenient method.

- *Quartz dryer*—A lightweight, hand-held dryer that sends out heat energy in the infrared spectrum.

- *Diffuser*—A nozzle attachment that goes on the end of a standard blow-dryer to shut off the air force but retain the heat for drying. It's heavier than the quartz dryer and more costly.

Hood dryers

Hood dryers are good for drying hair when you want to change its formation, as with straight hair that is damp set with rollers. This drying method is also useful for helping conditioner penetrate the hair. The hood should be large enough so that it fits over your head with room to place your hand between your head and the hood. Look for variable controls and a heavy, sturdy stand.

Towels

One hundred percent cotton, looped (not plush) towels are the best for drying hair. Or you can make a *drying mitt* by sewing together three sides of two facecloths to make a mitt. Make one mitt for each hand and connect them with a string for easy hanging.

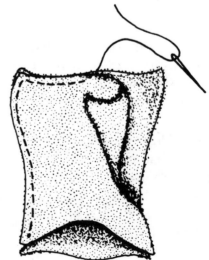

DRYING MITT

Hot rollers

The most effective tool to produce instant temporary curl. They vary in two ways: the *type of roller* (velvet covered, ribbed, spiked) and the *type of heat* (dry or mist).

The rollers—Spike rollers look like porcupines and can get tangled up in your hair. If you already have this kind of roller, remove the spikes by nipping off every other row with a razor or nail scissors. Slotted rollers don't tangle as easily. Clairol's Kindness slotted rollers are our favorite. They have an exclusive wax-filled inner core which gives you more gentle controlled heat for long-lasting body and curl. The new velvety-smooth-surfaced Clairol Custom CareRollers are terrific and promise no split ends from tangled roll-outs.

Dry versus mist sets—It really makes no difference which type you use. The heat from hot rollers does not damage hair, so there is no need to "replace" it with mist . . . nor does mist help "set" the curl any better.

Another variable to consider—the size of the unit. In general, the more you attempt to change the formation of your hair, the more rollers you need. You are the best judge of whether you need a five- or twenty-roller set.

Tips for styling—Experience is the best way to discover how long you need to keep the rollers in your hair to get the curl you want. Some hair might need only five minutes with rollers in; longer hair might need fifteen minutes. All hair types should wait two minutes after taking out the rollers for hair to cool before beginning to style it. End papers, or tissues cut into squares, are useful while rolling hair to avoid those scrunched-up ends we call "fishhooks." Some people erroneously believe these to be the result of heat damage. They're not. They're caused by ends that are not wound smoothly around the roller. Another tip: Buy extra prongs as soon as you buy a set of hot rollers . . . or send away for extras now if you already own a set. You are almost guaranteed to lose them at some point, so be prepared. Contact the store where you bought the rollers or the manufacturer to find out where to order more.

Curling irons

Curling irons give you the fastest, firmest temporary curl. Irons usually come in two diameters: The large iron is the most widely used to set the entire head; the small iron is used on ends of the hair. There are also irons that let you attach barrels of different diameters; however, these irons generally don't heat up as effi-

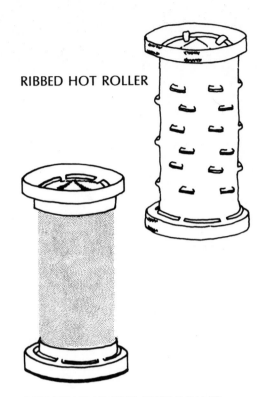

RIBBED HOT ROLLER

VELVETY-SMOOTH HOT ROLLER

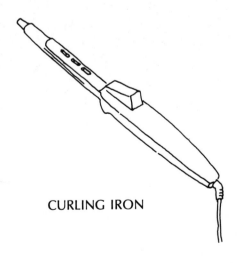

CURLING IRON

ciently as a central single iron. For those who are less dextrous, there are irons with a tip on the end so you can hold both ends as you rotate it. Whatever kind of curling iron you select, it should be thermostatically controlled, with a spring or manually operated blade hinge. As with hot rollers, mist curling irons are available, but we see no special advantage or disadvantage to them.

Tips for styling—Remember to clip hot "just-made" curls against your head until they cool. Also, curling irons can be used upside-down for shining and straightening hair.

Rollers

We set almost entirely on either dry or semidry hair, not on wet hair. Wet setting changes your hair's natural characteristics and is much more time-consuming than, for example, hot rollers, which use heat. For this reason, we view wet setting with rollers as a nearly outdated process. If you use rollers to set your hair, we recommend that you let it dry partially or entirely before using the rollers. The different types of rollers are as follows:

- *Plastic or nylon*—Not recommended for dry setting as they do not hold hair easily. If you choose to wet set your hair, try covering your nylon or plastic rollers with one-quarter-inch foam. Cut the foam into strips the size of the rollers and attach with Krazy Glue (rubber band over the seam will give good adhesion). Your rollers will be more luxurious and functional and will last longer. Secure rollers in hair with pins or picks.
- *Brush*—Not recommended as they tend to pull the hair and create a fuzzy effect on fine-textured hair.
- *Sponge*—Preferable to plastic or brush rollers as they are exceptionally kind to hair; however, it can be difficult to control the size of the curl you get with these rollers. Winding the soft sponge too tightly squashes the roller and you'll end up with a tight curl. Sponge rollers are best for long or finely textured hair.
- *Velcro*—Made of plastic covered with Velcro, which catches the hair and helps keep it in place. Velcro rollers give you exactly the right diameter of curl and are easier to use on dry hair than other rollers. They are especially good for short, fine hair.

Pins

All pins should have plastic tips on the ends and should be selected to match your hair color.

- *Bobby pins*—Use long ones when working with large sections of hair; small ones on fine hair.
- *Hairpins*—The thicker, longer ones are good for holding pincurls—or holding hot rollers in an emergency. The finer ones, called "invisible" pins, are used to secure ornamental effects.

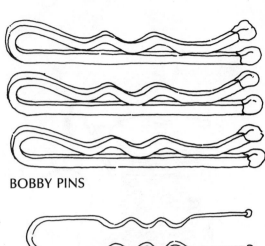

BOBBY PINS

Clips

These act as your "third hand" and are used for sectioning off hair and setting curls. They should not be sharp pointed and should grip all along the length. Double-pronged clips are easier to use than single; both plastic and metal clips work well. Clips come in two lengths: long, three or four inches, for holding large sections of hair; and short, two inches, for pincurls and holding strands of hair.

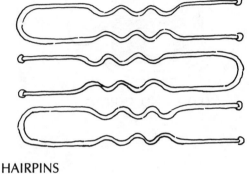

HAIRPINS

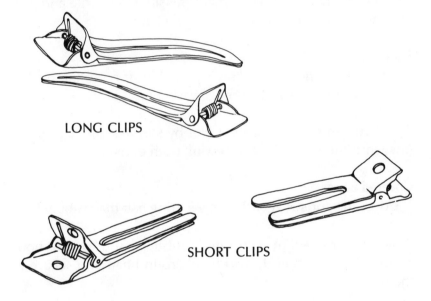

LONG CLIPS

SHORT CLIPS

Mist bottle

The least-used at home tool, but one of the most effective, especially for curly or permanented hair. Mist provides nature's helping hand—humidity—instantly. Use any type of mist that suits your style—from spraying plain water in an old glass-cleaner container to spraying mineral water out of a pretty glass apothecary bottle. It's a good idea to have an adjustable nozzle on the bottle so you can use a very fine mist to bring out curl or a heavy squirt when you want to wet down hair for setting or styling.

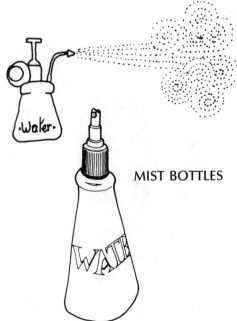

MIST BOTTLES

Styling—Fill a mist bottle with a mixture of half conditioner, half water, and spray it on any time your ends feel dry.

Clear plastic wrap

This is used to wrap the head when applying a conditioner that is left on the hair for approximately twenty minutes and rinsed out. The plastic helps hold body heat, which facilitates penetration of the conditioner throughout the hair.

Hairnet

A hairnet should be made of human hair, which camouflages better and is more elastic. Get the square flat type. To use for a chignon, lay the net over the length of the hair, twist it with the hair so it traps all the loose ends, then secure with hairpins.

Needle and thread

A large darning needle with a large eye and sewing thread the color of your hair can come in handy. Use them to secure hair ornaments and the ends of braids invisibly. A needle and thread are particularly helpful for styling fine hair.

Filet

This is also known as a "rat" . . . a filler for a rolled hairstyle. Make sure the one you select is washable.

Tip—You can make your own filet by stuffing one leg of pantyhose into the other leg and sewing both ends.

Covered bands

Covered bands are gentler for securing hair than rubber bands.

Tip—If you're caught with only a rubber band to use, hook a bobby pin to each end, twirl band around hair and secure with the pins.

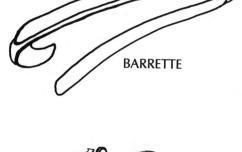

NEEDLE AND THREAD

BARRETTE

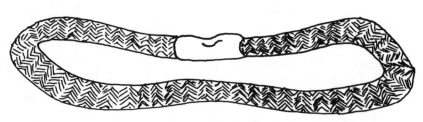

COVERED BAND

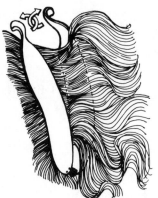

LONG-CLASP BARRETTE

Barrettes and Combs

These are ornaments that secure the hair (we call barrettes "slides" in England). A long-clasp barrette, used on long hair, gives a new, vertical line to a ponytail.

CHOOSING THE HAIR-CARE TOOLS
THAT ARE RIGHT FOR YOU

There are four different hair-styling possibilities: (1) You have wavy or curly hair and want a wavy or curly style or (2) you want a straight style; (3) you have straight hair and want a straight style or (4) you want a wavy or curly style.

What follows is a list of the four styling possibilities and the equipment each one requires for you to create the look you want. Looking at these four groups, you'll see immediately two truths about hair care. One: Long hair needs more equipment—and, consequently, more dexterity, time, and attention. Two: The more you try to change what nature has given you—opting for a straight hairstyle when you have curly hair, for instance—again, the more equipment, dexterity, time, and attention you'll need.

WAVY OR CURLY HAIR/WAVY OR CURLY STYLE

Wide-tooth comb, pick, mist bottle, Denman brush, lamp or quartz or diffusion dryer, short clips, hairdressing, spray shine.

For long hair add: bobby pins, hairpins, human-hair hairnet, long clips, needle and thread, barrettes, covered bands, filet.

WAVY OR CURLY HAIR/STRAIGHT STYLE

Wide-tooth comb, rattail comb, mist bottle, blow-dryer, large-diameter curling iron, Denman brush, flat-back brush, hair spray, short clips, long clips, hairdressing, spray shine, large- and small-diameter round brushes.

For long hair add: bobby pins, hairpins, human-hair hairnet, needle and thread, barrettes, covered bands, filet.

STRAIGHT HAIR/STRAIGHT STYLE

Wide-tooth comb, rattail comb, mist bottle, blow-dryer, Denman brush, flat-back brush, long clips, hairdressing, spray shine, antistatic material, barrettes.

For long hair, add: bobby pins, hairpins, human-hair hairnet, short clips, needle and thread, covered bands, ribbons.

STRAIGHT HAIR/WAVY OR CURLY STYLE

Wide-tooth comb, rattail comb, pick, mist bottle, hot rollers (not necessary if your hair is permed), blow-dryer (not necessary with a perm), lamp or quartz or diffusion dryer, curling iron (not necessary with a perm), flat-back brush, Denman brush, short clips, hairdressing, spray shine.

For long hair—or no perm—add: hot rollers, blow-dryer, curling iron, round brush, bobby pins, hairpins, human-hair hairnet, hair spray, needle and thread, covered bands, barrettes, ribbons.

9 YOUR HAIR, YOUR FACE, AND YOUR BODY

At this point, you have all the information you need to decide if a hairstyle suits your hair's natural characteristics, and you know the time you need to spend creating it, your skill level, and the equipment the style requires. You're just about ready to get the haircut you'll need for your style. Before you do, however, let's stop a moment to consider whether the hairstyle you've selected is a good choice for your *facial features* and your *body proportions*.

HOW A STYLE CAN HIDE OR HIGHLIGHT YOUR FEATURES

A hairstyle—the overall look of the style as well as the cut—can affect your facial features tremendously. Do you really know if the style you've selected from the hairstyle charts will be flattering to your eyes, your nose, your chin, the shape of your neck and back?

A hairstyle can *hide* those facial features you want to minimize, and it can also *highlight* those features you want to emphasize—or the ones you would prefer to hide. Analyze your face and then read the descriptions below so that when you make your final selection, you'll be sure you've chosen a style that will flatter your features as much as possible.

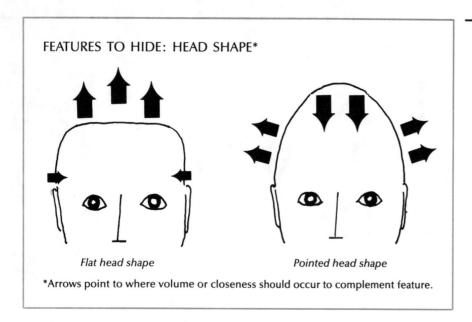

FEATURES TO HIDE: HEAD SHAPE*

Flat head shape   Pointed head shape

*Arrows point to where volume or closeness should occur to complement feature.

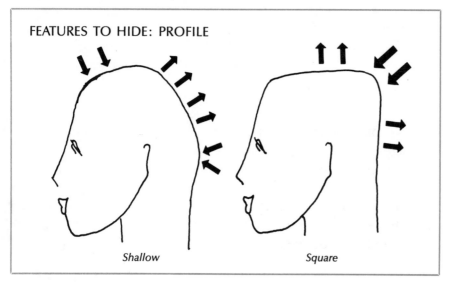

FEATURES TO HIDE: PROFILE

Shallow   Square

WHAT A STYLE CAN DO FOR YOUR FACE

Highlight: eyes, head shape, head size, nose, jaw, wide face, thin face, cheeks, ears, profile, neck, hairline, nape hairline, wide temples, narrow temples, hair's condition.

Hide: big ears, low nape hairline, high front hairline, large forehead, wide temples, narrow temples, sparse hair at the temples, low forehead, low hairline in front of ears, profile, head shape, jawline, neck shape, hair's condition.

Minimize: large chin or jaw, receding chin, wide face, long face, chubby cheeks.

Let's see how this works and what you should look for when trying to hide or highlight your features. First, gather all your hair away from your face (you may want to wet it) and look, really look, at yourself in a mirror—use two mirrors so you can get back and side views. Now find the sketch that best represents your features and see where the arrows point. These arrows show where hair should go to make the most, or the least, of the feature.

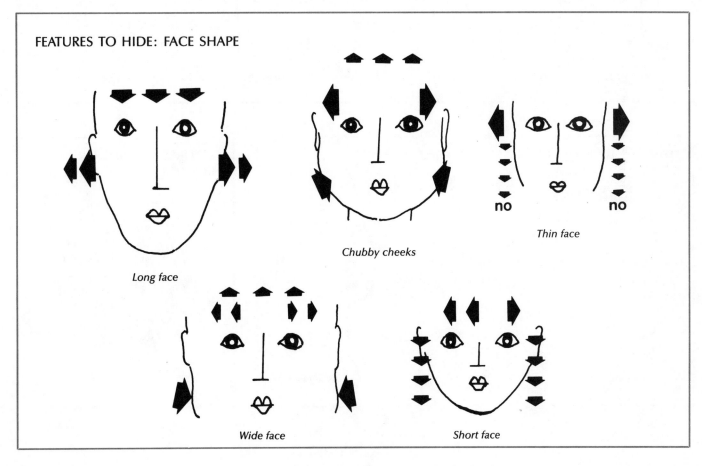

FEATURES TO HIDE: FACE SHAPE

Long face

Chubby cheeks

Thin face

no   no

Wide face

Short face

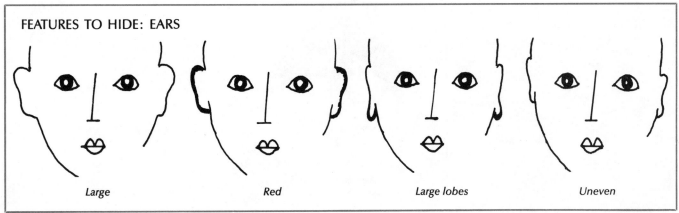

FEATURES TO HIDE: EARS

Large

Red

Large lobes

Uneven

FEATURES TO HIDE: NECK SHAPE

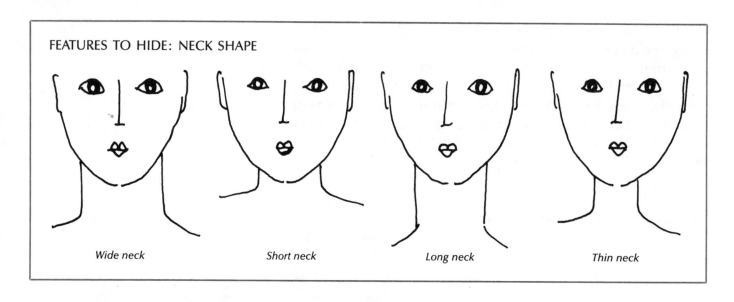

Wide neck   *Short neck*   *Long neck*   *Thin neck*

FEATURES TO HIDE: CHIN AND JAW LINES

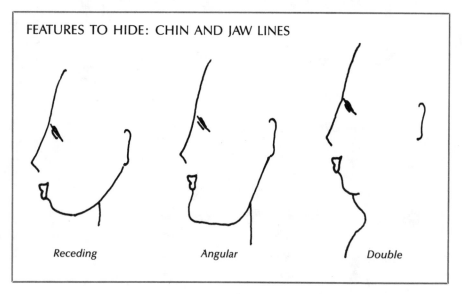

Receding   *Angular*   *Double*

FEATURES TO HIDE OR HIGHLIGHT: NAPE HAIRLINE

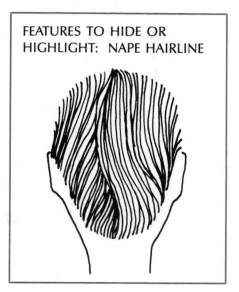

FEATURES TO HIGHLIGHT: FRONT HAIRLINE

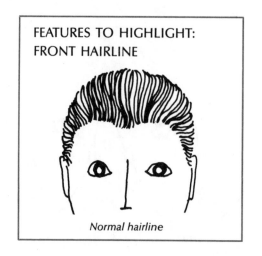

Normal hairline

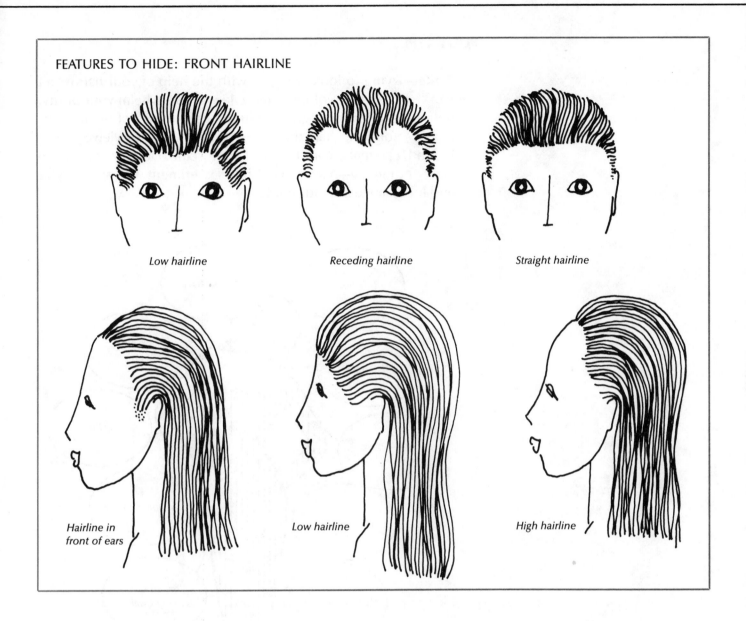

FEATURES TO HIDE: FRONT HAIRLINE

Low hairline   *Receding hairline*   *Straight hairline*

Hairline in front of ears   *Low hairline*   *High hairline*

THE BALANCE OF HAIR AND BODY

Besides making the most of your facial features, a hairstyle should be in balance with your overall body proportions.

Following are descriptions of the five basic types of women's bodies—*petite*, *small*, *medium*, *large*, and *tall*—and the characteristics of each type. How you wear your hair won't affect how the frame of your body looks, but it can affect how your shoulders, neck, and head size appear, which, in turn, affects your total appearance. The key words to keep in mind when considering if a hairstyle works with your body are "fullness" and "length."

BODY TYPE

Petite—Trying to look "bigger" with the help of your hair won't work. A long or a voluminous style will overwhelm your pretty, delicate proportions, giving you the appearance of being "top-heavy." Too-long hair that trails down the back, viewed from behind, can make your legs look minuscule. Don't try to change your petiteness—play it to the hilt. Experiment with short styles and let balance be your guide.

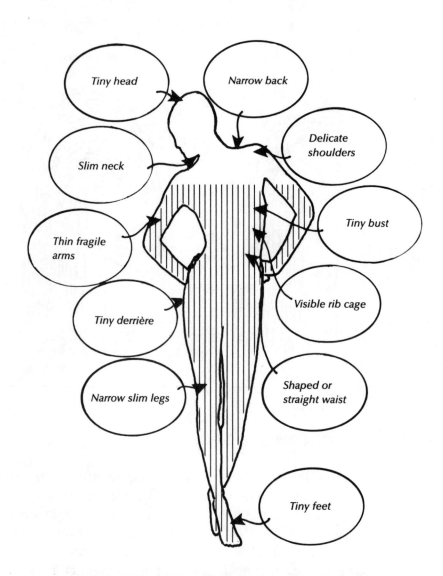

PETITE PROPORTIONS: Below 5'0". A TONED BODY, BOYISH "TWIGGY" FRAME. FRAGILE BODY STRUCTURE LIKE A BALLERINA.

Small—You fall between the "petite" and "medium" frames and should follow the guidelines for both categories. Don't overwhelm yourself with too much hair or "shorten" your appearance from the back with too long hair, and pay special attention to those features you want to hide or highlight.

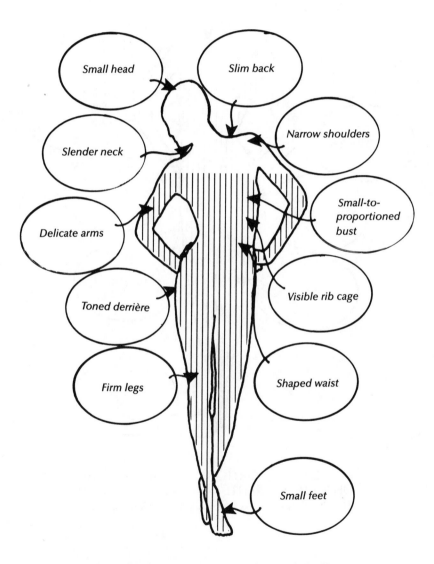

SMALL PROPORTIONS: 5'1" or 5'2". LARGER BONE STRUCTURE THAN "PETITE" BUT SMALLER THAN "MEDIUM."

Medium—You're fortunate because this shape gives you the most hairstyle options. Try what you like, and let considerations of hiding or highlighting features be your guide.

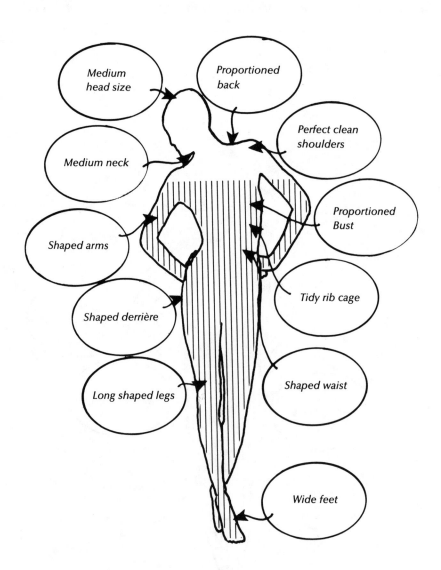

Medium head size

Proportioned back

Perfect clean shoulders

Medium neck

Proportioned Bust

Shaped arms

Tidy rib cage

Shaped derrière

Shaped waist

Long shaped legs

Wide feet

MEDIUM PROPORTIONS: 5'4" to 5'6". NOT AS DELICATE AS "PETITE" OR "SMALL," SHORTER THAN "TALL," AND SLIMMER THAN "LARGE."

Tall—A very short style can look extremely elegant, provided you carry it off with good posture. You can also carry off long and full hair magnificently. Just be careful hair doesn't look untidy or busy—simple elegance is you at your best.

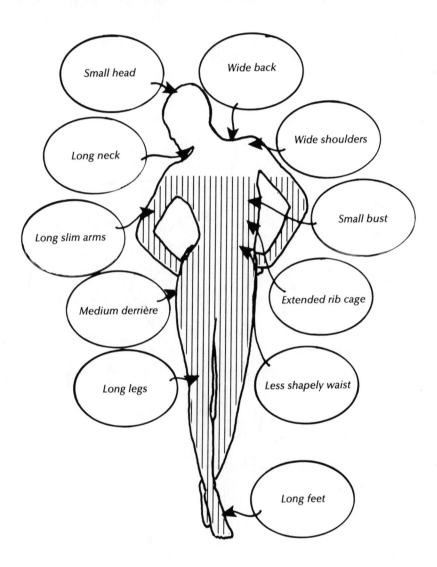

TALL PROPORTIONS: 5'7" or above.

Large—Too short a style can make you look like a turtle peeking out of its shell. Even though short hair can be practical, a short *flat* style can highlight how big you are. If you're not blessed with an abundance of hair with which to create an expanded style, you might consider getting a permanent. Remember, though, don't go overboard with length—a style that's too long and full will make you look twice your size. Keep balance in mind when playing off fullness against length.

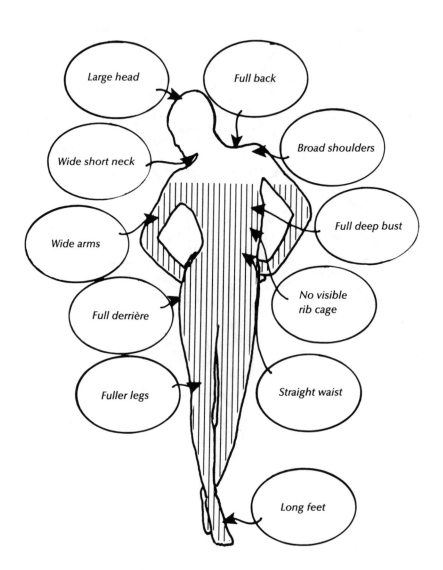

LARGE PROPORTIONS: ANY HEIGHT.

10 THE HAIRCUT— KEY TO THE PERFECT HAIRSTYLE

The last variable you need to know before you make your hairstyle selection is how your hair should be *cut* to get the style you want.

The haircut is a crucial step in creating your perfect hairstyle. A good cut makes all the difference between a hairstyle that looks neat and one that looks sloppy, and it can go a long way toward enhancing your best features and minimizing your worst ones. The haircut consists of two parts: (1) *Design lines* (or exterior lengths)—the line of the hair as it hangs all around the face and head; and (2) *Layering*—the graduation of length within the design line, which can range from no layering at all to layering all over the head.

In this chapter, we give examples and illustrations of all the different possibilities for design lines and layering and tell you which facial features each design line and type of layering flatter, which body proportions they emphasize or minimize, and which lines and layers are best for the quality of your hair. Each of the forty hairstyle charts includes a sketch of the haircut you'll need to get the style pictured. Compare the haircut sketch on the chart with the information in this chapter to be certain you've selected a hairstyle that will suit you perfectly.

DESIGN LINES

There are three kinds of design lines—*front* lines, *side* lines, and *back,* or nape, lines. Look at the bold black lines on the illustrations to see what each of the different design lines will do for you. By understanding design lines, you'll know whether you should have bangs, if short or long hair is a better bet for you, and so on.

Specific directions for design lines are included on each of the hairstyle charts as well as instructions for how to modify the design lines you've selected to get the cut you need for the style you select. Be sure to show the sketch of the design lines to your hairdresser so he or she can give you exactly the cut you need.

Front Lines

There are four basic front design lines:

Horizontal line—This line is straight-across bangs. They should never be cut too short—never shorter than the brows as they will add pounds to your features. Try not to wear them too "perfect"—tousle them just a bit with your fingers for the best look. This bang is usually best for straight hair.

FRONT: HORIZONTAL LINES

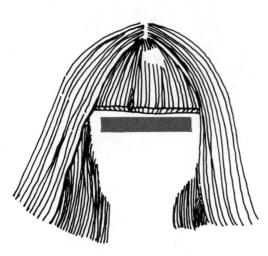

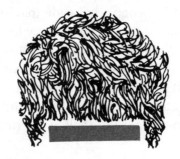

Curved line—This line is good for women with prominent temples as it helps slim the width across the forehead. Curved bangs are generally cut close to the eyes, so your brows will be covered. If you select this line, use makeup to really emphasize your eyes and bring them out—otherwise they may "disappear" under the bangs.

FRONT: CURVED LINES

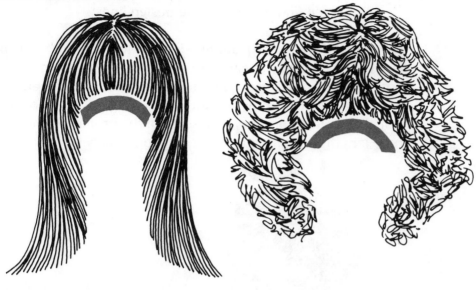

FRONT: "V" LINES

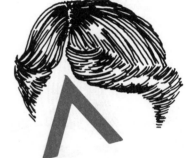

"V" line—This shape is usually not apparent when you first look because the hair turns or folds off the face, disguising the V. To roll the hair away from the face, you must have dexterity with a brush and a blow-dryer, curling iron, or hot rollers. These front lengths are generally long—from brow- to chin-length. A wavy or curly formation will help in the effort to keep them off the face. Since the "V" line is full and adds lift, it's a great disguiser of facial features.

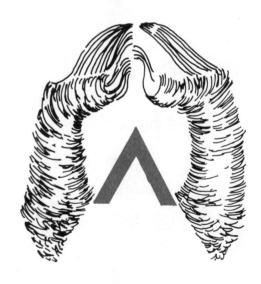

Hairline line—This frames the hairline and is generally used for lengths no longer than the bridge of the nose and as short as a quarter inch from your hairline, it's also the line that results from having no bangs at all. If the hair at your temples is sparse, this line may not be for you as it will expose them. It's a good choice, however, for any woman who wants a short and practical line with no hair against her face. It highlights your nose, jaw, face shape, cheeks—in short, all of your features.

FRONT: HAIRLINE LINES

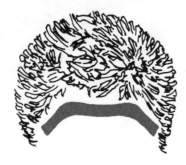 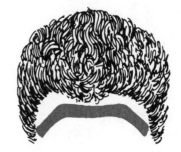

Side Lines

Again, you'll find four basic side design lines:

Horizontal line—This square line is used to "perk up" a shape, and can just cover the ear or extend all the way down to your bottom. It is usually cut quite precisely—hair perfect—and will work on all hair textures and formations. If it is long enough, it will hide cheekbones, jaw, and some of the profile. However, to have length with this line you need good-quality hair.

SIDES: HORIZONTAL LINES

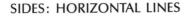

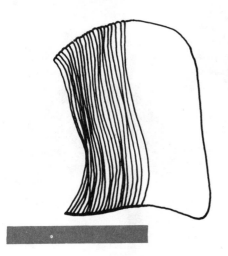

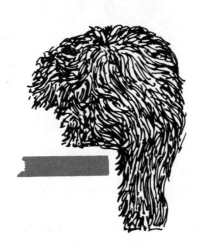

Diagonal line (I)—This line, which starts short in front and gets longer in the back, is probably the most popular side design line. It is usually used in conjunction with the front V design line. It exposes the cheeks, but removes heavy hair weight and softens the hair around the hairline. This line combines the practicality of short hair around the face with hair that's long enough to cover the ears, chin, or neckline, and can be worn long or short.

SIDES: DIAGONAL LINES (I)

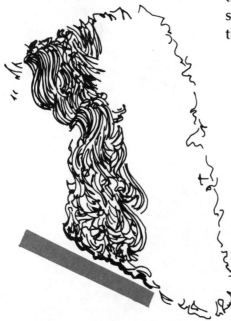

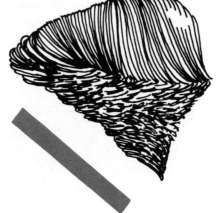

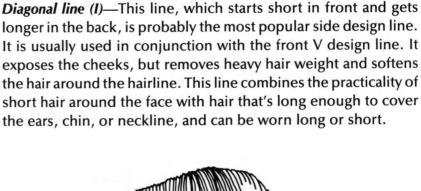

60

Diagonal line (II)—This diagonal starts long in front and gets shorter in the back. You have to be careful with this one because it can look contrived if the slant is too pronounced. It was a very popular line in the early 1960s—part of the swinging blunt cuts that worked so well with miniskirts—because it gives hair a lot of weight so it swings around the face. This line should be cut with a *slight,* never an acute, angle. If you have poor posture—slightly hunched shoulders, high shoulders, or a neck that bends forward—this line can remove weight from your back and perk up the look of your posture, while the longer side lengths toward the front can disguise the jawbones, cheekbones, and profile. It will, in short, create an illusion of lengthening the neck while hiding the profile.

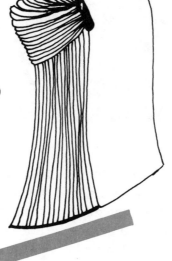

SIDES: DIAGONAL LINES (II)

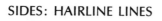

Hairline line—Again, be careful with this line, because the shorter the sides are, the more perfect or prettier your ears must be. A natural-looking, slightly casual approach to cutting and shaping is important for this line; a very perfect precision cut would tend to make you look as though you'd just stepped out of the barber shop. This is a totally practical line . . . but the shorter your hair goes, remember, the more your features are exposed.

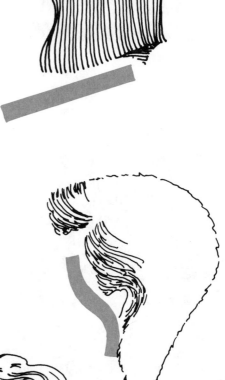

SIDES: HAIRLINE LINES

Back Lines

There are four back design line possibilities:

Horizontal line—This line covers the back hairline and is usually used for longer lengths of hair. The line is excellent for maintaining long hair, especially if your hair is fine and fragile, as it requires frequent trims to keep smart looking. This line can give a lift to the profile and highlight the condition of your hair.

BACK: HORIZONTAL LINES

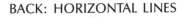

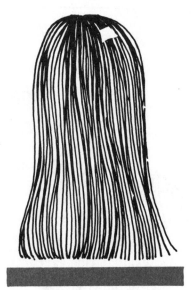

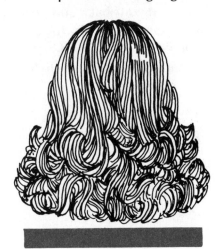

"V" line—This line is probably the most popular nape line because it allows short, practical lengths around the face with length down the middle. It is excellent for a woman with a wide neck and shoulders as the line covers the neck and breaks up the shoulders with a trail of hair down the middle of the neck and back. Be sure the line is cut so that the V does not stick out as you move your head.

BACK: "V" LINES

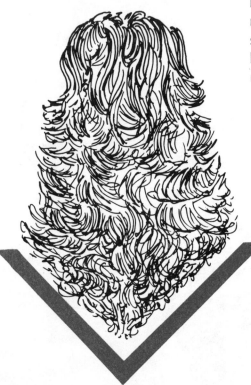

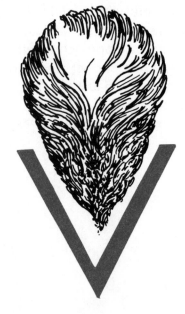

Curved line—This line is generally used on longer lengths of hair to cover the hairline. It can perk up your look because it removes heavy length from the back of the neck; it also enables you to have hair at the sides of your head or behind the ears, which is soft and flattering. It can add pounds to the shoulders and neck, however, when viewed from behind. It can also look too contrived if the shape is too curved. With this line, "less is more," so take care that the line is not too curved.

BACK: CURVED LINES

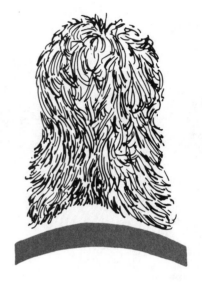

Hairline line—This line is used on short hair—from short to very short. The shorter your hair, the more hair weight is removed and the more the growth direction takes over, exposing all those funny little cowlicks around the hairline. If your hair grows straight up at the back or if you have a low or peculiar hairline shape, those factors are going to predominate if you select this line and your hair is cut very short. On the other hand, the shorter your hair, the more practical it can be. This line should not be hard, sharp, or severe, but soft, as if nature grew it rather than a hairdresser cut it.

BACK: HAIRLINE LINES

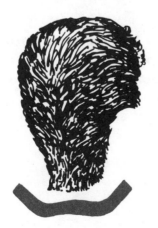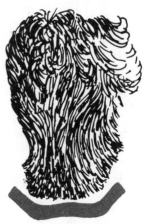

LAYERING

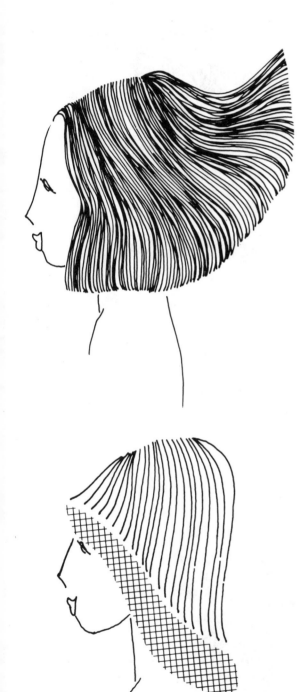

Layering is the key for making hair fuller or flatter. The number of layers, where they are put and where not, whether you have some, a lot, or none at all, determines how your hairstyle works and falls into shape. Most women wonder whether they should have layers in their hair or not—this decision should be made *after* you have decided which design lines suit your face and features.

Following are descriptions of the seven different types of layering that will help you decide what kind of layering—if any—you should have. The sketches that accompany these descriptions also appear on the hairstyle charts. Each chart includes special directives to tell you and your hairdresser how to modify these seven key cuts for the particular style you select.

1. No layers—This is excellent for fine, thin hair, provided the quality of the hair is good and holds up as it grows in length, not becoming brittle or split. The hair looks lovely and swings and moves easily. The major problem with no layers is that as women with fine hair grow their hair, they do not always follow a regime of careful conditioning, shampooing, combing, and using implements correctly. The result: hair that wears out so it looks terrible. If that happens, try layering and read on. If, however, you have thin, fine hair but it is in good condition, we often recommend that you keep it blunt and all one length. No need to try layers—you'll be fine. Women with coarse-textured hair, particularly if it is also wavy, require layering to help control the volume.

This *hides:* big ears, low nape line, high front hairline, low hairline in front of the ears, profile, head shape, jawline neckshape.

This *highlights:* thin faces, your hair's condition.

2. The best of both worlds: the luxury of length combined with the practicality of layers—This is a good cut for women who want length but don't want their hair to just hang, as can happen with no layering. The layering here gives you some softness, can remove weight, and can make the ends work for your hair to lift it.

Just a small amount of layering around the design line can be very flattering and soft. This is an example of long layers on the top, which create smoothness, and layering around the bottom so that you have little pieces of hair to soften the face. It still covers the ears, can be long enough to touch the shoulders, but has layering to prevent the back from just hanging down in a big flop of hair.

This *hides:* big ears, low nape line, profile, head shape.

This *highlights:* your hair's condition.

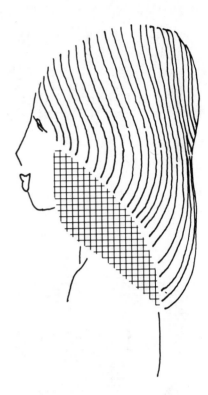

3. The hair is almost all one length, with only a small amount of layering from the chin to the shoulders, producing tiny wisps around the face—You can use a hot roller set with this cut to get a lot of curl, particularly if your hair is the right texture, formation, and quantity. This cut is good for most hair textures, except very, very curly hair.

This *hides:* big ears, low nape line, high front hairlines, large forehead, wide temples, low hairline in front of the ears, sparse hair at the temples, head shape, jawline, neck shape, thin face, chubby cheeks. . . . It's a great disguiser.

This *highlights:* hair condition.

4. An extremely popular short haircut that's easy to care for, practical, and suits a broad range of hair characteristics—(You may recognize this cut as the one Princess Diana has.) The layers around the face and neck shorten the hair so that it flips and turns attractively; the crown, left longer, leaves the hair smooth—you have smoothness on the top with softness all the way around the face. Also, it leaves a weight of hair at the back of the head so you don't feel as though all your hair is shaved off. The cut disguises head proportions—if you have a flat or pointed head, that extra length at the back will fill it in. The sides should cover the ears, the layering should be to the top of the ears, and the bangs should be cut anywhere from the eyelid to the tip of the nose (and flipped to the sides).

This *hides:* ears, low nape line, high front hairline, large forehead, wide temples, low hairline in front of the ears, sparse hair at the temples, low forehead, narrow temples, profile, head shape.

This *highlights:* hair condition, nose, jaw, cheeks, neck.

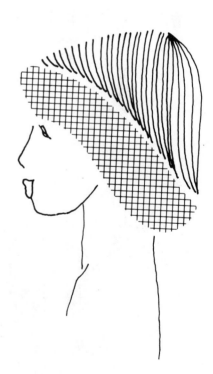

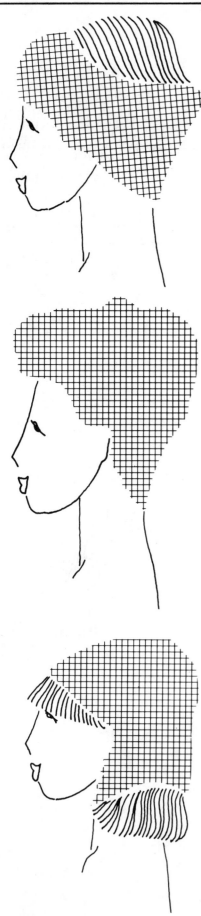

5. The perfect cut for women who are nervous about going too short but who don't have the quantity or texture of hair, or the skill, to keep longer hair—About two-thirds of the head has an extensive amount of layering, while the crown is a longer length which gives the cut a smooth look. The layering around the face adds softness and those nice wispy ends. This is a good cut for women who opt for short hair.

This *hides:* ears, high front hairline, large forehead, wide temples, low hairline in front of the ears, sparse hair at the temples, low forehead, hair condition, profile, head shape.

This *highlights:* nose, jaw, face shape, neck, nape line.

6. All-over layering—This cut covers a broad range of hairstyles. Whatever style is chosen, however, there are key points to remember. Many women have hair that seems to come to a point when it is cut—the width is level with the ears rather than being above the eyes. When this happens—width and no height on top—it tends to make you look plump, so be sure there is some width above the eyes. The layering can be done so that when the hair's length and weight are removed, its formation, texture, and quantity work together to give it a lift and make it look fuller and bigger. If it's done well, all-over layering can help enhance your features and can look perfectly fine even on needle-straight hair. Done poorly, it can exaggerate all your worst features and look dreadful. Be sure to get a good haircut.

This *hides:* hair condition, high front hairline, sparse hair at the temples, low forehead, profile, and head shape.

This *highlights:* nose, jaw, face shape, cheeks, chin, ears, neck, hairline in front of the ears.

7. A mixture of everything: layering all over the head, but with length in the bangs and the nape of the neck—The layering lifts the hair and gives it volume, while the bangs and the nape, which are heavier and bulkier, allow you to disguise more of your features. This cut is particularly good for women whose hair grows in a low or peculiar direction, as it helps hold the hair down and look neater.

This *hides:* low nape hairline, high front hairline, large forehead, wide temples, low hairline in front of the ears, sparse hair at the temples, low forehead, narrow temples, profile, head shape, jawline, neck, hair condition—it's a great disguiser.

This *highlights:* wide face, ears (if cut to expose them).

Now you will be ready to select your perfect hairstyle!

11 HOW TO FIND THE PERFECT HAIRDRESSER

After you've selected your perfect hairstyle from the charts, how do you find a hairdresser to give you the cut, perm, or other hair-care maintenance you require—in short, how do you find the perfect hairdresser? The perfect hairdresser is one you feel comfortable with, can talk to easily, and, most important, one who gives you the results you want! How do you go about finding this person?

The first thing to do is get recommendations. Ask friends whose hairstyles you admire whom they go to. But don't limit yourself just to friends. Anyone you see anywhere with great-looking hair is a source for a recommendation. Don't be intimidated about asking a stranger who her hairdresser is; most women are flattered to be told their hair looks terrific. Some places to be sure to keep your eyes open for great-looking hair and a good recommendation are:

- your favorite boutique
- your favorite restaurant
- health clubs, tennis clubs, country clubs
- in short, places you enjoy going to, places that reflect your personal style and taste, places women who are concerned with the way they look might frequent

More excellent sources for recommendations are:

- the beauty or style editor of your local newspaper
- the director of your local modeling agency
- an airline training or grooming center
- an amateur theater group

You don't have to live in New York or Los Angeles to find a top-notch salon. There are many, many excellent salons in every part of the country, in small towns as well as big ones. One of the best, in our opinion, is in Atlanta. You know it's a top-level operation from the minute you walk in the door and feel the atmosphere—light, airy, understated, and attractive. The staff is pleasant, efficient . . . and informed. They are constantly on the move, traveling to New York and the West Coast to attend seminars, trade shows, and training programs that keep them abreast of the latest in hair care and hairstyles. They travel frequently to Europe—not just for training programs, but to attend the fashion shows as well, to see the latest trends in fashion and hairstyles the moment they first come down the runway.

One very good way to tell if a salon is a good one is to simply look around you. Are there pictures of hairstyles on the wall? Someone has gone to the trouble to select, pay for, and hang these pictures and, in our experience, they are a dead giveaway of the taste level of the salon's operators. What's on the counter tops? If they are filled with hair spray and rollers, it's a clue the salon is not practicing the latest techniques. Is there a style book—a book filled with pictures of the salon's favorite hairstyles? It should reflect the kind of hairstyles the operators are currently doing. Finally, how does the staff's hair look? Hairdressers are in the beauty business by choice, and are walking advertisements of their own capability and taste. Pay special attention to the receptionist's hair—it should epitomize the salon's work.

Another factor to consider: *price.* Ask the receptionist for a price list (you may feel more comfortable telephoning from home). Be specific. You may be told that a cut is, say, $15, but end up paying a bill for $25 because you forgot to ask if shampooing, conditioning, and blow-drying were included in the price of the cut or additional charges.

As with most things in life, you usually get what you pay for. If the price is high, the level of quality should be high, too. A salon has to take in so much money to keep going. If it has many clients, it can keep prices down . . . but those clients may be rushed in and rushed out, and not receive very much attention. Ask the receptionist how many clients per hour each stylist services. If the answer is three or more, you can be pretty sure that you will not be given much attention. Look for a salon where the operators spend more time with each client, taking only one or two per hour. The salon may have to charge more, but the operators will take the time to do better work.

A word of caution—beware of salons that are constantly

advertising sales. They must be doing something wrong if they have to seek clients by this method.

MAKING AN APPOINTMENT

The best time to make a first appointment is usually in the beginning of the week, before the salon's midweek/weekend rush. If a particular hairdresser has been recommended to you, ask specifically for him or her—don't be pressured into accepting an appointment with someone else on the staff who may not be as busy. It is worth the wait, and don't be afraid to say so. Ask about coming in for a free five- or ten-minute consultation in which you meet the hairdresser and discuss what you want done. This is an excellent way to find out what you are getting into, but, unfortunately, only about 10 percent of salons agree to do this with any regularity. If you cannot get a consultation, tell the receptionist the name of the person who recommended you and explain what you want done. The receptionist will be able to communicate this to the hairdresser, briefing him or her on what to expect from you.

Your first appointment is really a kind of trial run, and so it's a wise idea to start with the simplest of services—a trim, perhaps, or a blow-dry. Nothing drastic. You have to build a trust with the hairdresser before asking him or her to make a major change with your hair.

When you arrive for your first appointment, there are some things you can do to be a good client and start things off right:

- Be on time.
- Leave children and pets at home . . . It's much more relaxing for you as well as for the salon.
- Wear the makeup and outfit that best reflect your taste.
- When you meet the hairdresser, offer your hand in greeting and look him or her squarely in the eye—hairdressers spend most of their day talking into mirrors and appreciate this direct personal contact.
- Show the hairdresser the photo of the hairstyle you've selected from the charts in this book and, if appropriate, the cutting sketch.
- Use the shampooing session as an opportunity to do more research—ask the shampooer what products he or she is using, why they were selected, and what they would recommend for your particular type of hair.
- Ask the hairdresser if you can help out by handing things.

- Don't read, fidget, or turn around to talk—the hairdresser positions your head in a particular way for a reason.
- Don't intimidate your hairdresser with your attitude—by talking about the others in his field who have worked on your hair.

As you are being served, judge the hairdresser on his or her concentration, consideration, dexterity (does he or she make clean partings?), hygiene, and personal appearance. See if at the end of your session the stylist offers information on how to look after your hair and explains the tools you will need for maintenance and how to use them.

When the styling is completed, don't be afraid to examine the results. Use a hand mirror to check out the front, side, and back views. If you like what you see—smile, say thanks, shake hands . . . and tip. Here's what we suggest: 15 percent of the total cost to the stylist if he or she does any or all of the following—cutting, coloring, permanenting, shampooing, blow-drying. If there is an individual who does nothing but shampoo your hair, tip $1 . . . and if there is someone who does just the blow-drying, tip $1 to $2.

If you are not pleased with the results, or with any aspect of the service, don't be afraid to tell the hairdresser and, if need be, the manager or salon owner. Then start looking elsewhere.

If you are pleased, set up an appointment for the cut you need for the hairstyle you have selected. *Be sure to bring this book with you so the stylist can see the photograph of the hairstyle you want and follow the cutting guides—and, if necessary, the suggestions for permanents or coloring.*

You're at the start of a happy relationship with your hairdresser. To help maintain it, know how to communicate with him or her. If you understand your hair and the language your hairdresser uses, you have a better chance of avoiding any confusion and misunderstanding . . . and getting exactly the results you want.

12 HOW TO TALK TO YOUR HAIRDRESSER

If you go into a salon and ask for a "blunt cut," thinking you are asking for a cut like a "bob," you are headed for trouble—big trouble. Blunt cut simply means the technique of using scissors, rather than a razor, to cut the hair bluntly at the tips; a "layered" haircut can be "blunt cut." If what you envisioned was a haircut of one even length, you ask for a "bob."

There are a few terms that crop up again and again in hairdressing, and it's a good idea to learn them and what they mean so you can make yourself understood, and so you can easily understand just what your hairdresser is suggesting for your hair before it's too late.

It would be fabulous if there were a universal basic hairdressing language. It would enable a woman to walk into any salon, anyplace she might be traveling, and ask for and get precisely what she wants. We have tried to establish a universal tongue in our training program, which reaches thousands of salons around the world, and we're going to give you here the terms most commonly used and accepted in most salons across the country.

Following, you'll find definitions of the key words that will help you and your hairdresser communicate. We've arranged them in a progression, taking you from the words you'll want to use in an initial consultation or meeting to the cutting stage and the finishing or styling process. Learn them and use them and you're on the way to a happy salon experience . . . and to getting exactly the results you want.

Consultation Terminology

These are the words to use when you first talk to your hairdresser, so you can establish the type of service you want:

No change—Helping maintain what you've got . . . with a shampoo, conditioning treatment, or styling.

Slight change—A trim on the top, sides, or back; a new parting; reshaped bangs; a fuller style; a smaller style; a temporary color.

Temporary change—A special do (braiding, chignon, rolling, folding) for a special occasion.

Total permanent change—Changing the length, texture, formation, or color of hair.

Repair—Correcting the cut, perm, color, or hair condition.

Restyle—Total reshaping of hairstyle.

Trim—Cutting a small amount of hair (bangs, length, back of neck) to tidy hair, maintaining the existing hairstyle.

Virgin hair—Hair not previously treated with tints, lighteners, or permanents.

Falling point—The natural point from which hair is distributed.

Temporary style—A style where the longevity relies on your ability to avoid the elements and experiences of everyday life: rain, sleeping, sports.

Minimum Care style—A style that works easily for you, your hair, and how you live . . . chosen through an understanding of your hair's unique texture, quantity, and formation.

Cutting Terminology

Next are the key words to know about cutting:

Scissors—The tool most used for precision haircutting for contemporary hairstyles.

Razor—The tool most used to thin or point hair.

Blunt cut—A type of cut achieved using scissors.

Tapered cut—A type of cut achieved using a razor or thinning shears.

Bob—A one-length haircut.

Graduation—A layered haircut.

Subtle graduation—Selective or limited use of layers.

General graduation—All-over layering.

Original partings and sections—The basic lines that divide the head in preparation for cutting.

Reference points—Corners of eyes, brows, lips, nose, chin, neck, shoulders.

Design line—The initial line cut to define proportion and shape of style.

Guidelines—Already-cut hair sections.

Holding position and angle—The degree of direction hair is combed and positioned for cutting.

Pruning—The subtle creation of different lengths of hair, using the tips of scissors, to give hairstyle a softer, slightly disheveled effect.

Notching—Cutting hair on the design line, usually around the face, with scissors in a way that resembles pinking shears, to give a slightly uneven look.

Finishing Terminology

The following are words to use after your hair's been cut but before it's completely styled:

Blow-dry—Use of a hand-dryer in combination with hands or brush to remove moisture from hair by air force and to temporarily increase or decrease volume in the hair. Used on Minimum Care hairstyles to encourage hair's natural tendencies—especially formation (referred to as "form drying")—or to remove natural tendencies (called "force drying").

Lamp dry—Use of still, stationary heat to encourage natural or chemical curl.

Diffusion dry—Addition of an appliance (a diffuser) to the end of a blow-dryer to shut down the wind force but retain heat for the same result as lamp drying.

Hot, or thermal, set—Use of a heated appliance (hot rollers, curling iron) for the fastest way to temporarily change hair formation by curling hair, adding volume, and for temporarily shining hair to improve quality.

13 THE BEST PRODUCTS FOR YOUR HAIR

Once you have found your perfect hairstyle, you need to know just what to do to keep it looking its best for as long as possible—in short, what products you should use on your hair and how you should use them so they work most effectively. If you are puzzled about which shampoos are best for your type of hair; the difference between a creme rinse and conditioner and if you need to use either; when to use a setting lotion and when to use a hair spray . . . you'll find the answers here—and more. We think you'll find some surprises, too—some new and unexpectedly effective ways of caring for your hair, making it more manageable, more lustrous than it's ever been before!

The Products

Shampoo—A foaming cleanser for the hair and scalp. Many come formulated for dry hair (containing a high amount of fatty acids), oily hair (minimum amount of fatty acids), or dandruff (containing sulfur or zinc pyrithione). In general, the more a nonformulated shampoo foams and sudses, the more suitable it is for oily hair (nonformulated shampoos may be too strong for dry hair, causing static).

Creme rinse—A lotion that removes tangles by leaving a residue on the hair. Using creme rinse is like waxing a car—it leaves a shine but doesn't do the metal any good.

Conditioner—These range from the "instant" variety, which remove tangles, to the deep penetrating treatments, which require heat and take twenty to thirty minutes to restructure damaged hair shafts before being rinsed out of the hair. Some conditioners are designed to be left on the hair, particularly balsam or protein products, which coat the hair shaft, and placenta conditioners, which neutralize the high acidity level and dryness of damaged hair, especially hair that has been colored.

Setting lotion—A gel or liquid applied to wet hair to create a shape, especially to give support to fine hair or control the formation of curly hair. Liquids can be diluted with water to adjust their strength. The favorite of professionals: Tenax.

Hairdressing—An oil or creme to add temporary shine and luster to hair and to control static. Should be used in moderation.

Spray shine—A lanolin spray used sparingly to give hair shine.

Hair spray—Used to hold hair in shape. Most hair sprays come in hard-to-hold or normal formulas. Whichever you choose, look for a spray that's fast-drying, fine misting, water-soluble, not heavily perfumed, and combable, nonflaky and nondusty when dry. Test by spraying into the palm of your hand. If the mist looks shiny or feels tacky, it's too strong. Hair spray should be used moderately; overuse of spray will dull hair.

HOW TO USE THE PRODUCTS

If Your Hair Is Oily

Oily hair is caused by an oily scalp—a scalp with sebaceous glands working overtime producing oil. The oil wends its way down the hair shaft—particularly if hair is thin and fine—making it a "greasy magnet" for attracting dirt and grime. Sometimes, however, particularly if hair is coarse and curly, the oils do not trickle down the hair shaft, and an oily scalp is accompanied by dry hair.

To treat an oily scalp and oily hair—Use a shampoo designed for oily hair, sudsing with warm water and rinsing with cool water to help close pores temporarily. Rinse hair with a mixture of one cup cool water and one tablespoon cider vinegar or strained lemon juice—work some of it into the scalp, too. This mildly acidic rinse will remove any remaining traces of soap or oil that may be coating the hair. Avoid creme rinses and conditioners.

To help remove tangles—Use a wide-tooth comb and the force of water from a shower head to assist you . . . or apply a watered-down creme rinse or conditioner just on the ends or tangled sections of your hair.

To treat an oily scalp and dry ends—Use an oily-hair-formula shampoo. Place it in a bottle with a long nozzle, and aim the shampoo along the scalp. Lather the scalp. Rinse with cool water. Condition the ends or dry portion of your hair with a creme rinse or conditioner.

If Your Hair Is Dry

Dry hair can be caused by: an inability of the sebaceous glands to produce sufficient natural oils; the normal slowing down of this oil production with age; an inability of naturally produced oils to wend their way from the scalp down the hair shaft, particularly if hair is coarse or curly; the effects of the elements—wind, sun; the effects of chemicals—coloring, straightening, permanents.

To treat dry but not damaged hair—Use a shampoo for dry hair and follow with an instant conditioner or creme rinse every time you shampoo. Once a week, use a protein or balsam conditioner to coat the hair shaft and help it hold onto its supply of water and oil.

To control flyaway hair—Rub a bit of hairdressing oil or creme on your palms and work into the hair. Restore shine with spray shine.

If Your Hair Is Damaged

If abuse by the environment, chemicals, or misuse of appliances has structurally damaged your hair, there are ways to improve its appearance temporarily. Unfortunately, however, nothing short of removing the damage with a pair of scissors and letting your hair grow out can actually repair badly damaged hair.

To temporarily improve damaged hair—Use balsam conditioners, protein conditioners, or deep-penetrating restructuring conditioners frequently.

To condition color-treated hair—Use placenta conditioners to neutralize the acidity level.

You might also try this home remedy: Warm some mayonnaise in a saucepan. Apply it to hair and scalp with a paintbrush. Wrap the head with a hot, damp towel, and cover with foil. Wait twenty minutes, then remove wrap. Wash out mayonnaise with mild shampoo, and rinse hair with cool water. Your hair should be considerably shinier and more manageable.

If You Have Dandruff

Dandruff can be caused by a variety of factors, including excessively strong substances in contact with the scalp, poor health, medications, and stress. There are two types of dandruff: oily, which clings to the scalp, and dry, which flakes off easily, falling down the hair shaft and onto your neck and clothes, and can sometimes occur as a byproduct of aging.

To treat oily dandruff—Brush your hair gently and frequently to assist loosening the dandruff scales. Wash with a medicated shampoo—one containing sulfur or zinc pyrithione—making sure you get the shampoo on the scalp and not just in the hair. You may feel that your dandruff is getting worse after trying this treatment, but you are really succeeding in loosening the dandruff scales from the scalp—the first step toward their removal.

To treat dry dandruff—Wash hair with a creamy, fatty-rich shampoo, and massage the scalp with your fingertips frequently to stimulate the sebaceous glands to produce more oil.

WHAT EVERYONE SHOULD DO—EXPERIMENT!

Your hair goes through changes—as the seasons change, as you travel from one climate to another, as your body goes through its monthly cycle or reacts to stress caused by illness or emotional strains. At these times, you may find you need to experiment with different products until your hair returns to its usual condition. The most sensible way to experiment is to buy small, sample-size bottles of the products you think might do the trick and try them until you hit the combination that suits you best.

14 TRANSITION HAIR:

HOW TO GROW OUT WHAT YOU DON'T LIKE

Growing out hair—whether you're attempting to grow out the length, layers, bangs, a permanent, or a coloring process—can be a lengthy process. To see yourself through to the end, you're going to need some patience. The tips we give below will help you handle your hair as it grows out so it will look attractive . . . and so you'll have the psychological motivation to stick with your goal until you realize it.

GROWING OUT LENGTH

Even though you're trying to grow your hair longer, you still need to visit your hairdresser for trims to keep it tidy. One mistake that can occur: You go to your hairdresser for a slight trim and end up with a major haircut that sets you back months. The reason for this is usually poor communication. Let your hairdresser know you are not looking for the perfect haircut or style at this point but simply an interim look.

Some illusion tricks to help you while you're growing out the length:

- Lift up the sides of your hair and secure them with barrettes, combs, or a headband. You'll reveal the back lengths of your hair and the total effect will automatically appear longer.
- Try a permanent. It will increase your hair's volume and create the look and feel of more hair.

- Look at the hairstyle charts and photographs and select a brand-new interim style—one that's a little longer than the length you presently have so you can "grow" into it.

GROWING OUT LAYERS

All the tips for growing out length will help you here, especially getting a permanent. A permanent not only increases the volume of your hair, it also hides a multitude of sins. When you are growing out layers, your hair can quickly lose shape and look untidy. Perms are great for helping to mask the unevenness in layers that results.

Other tips:

- Set hair with hot rollers. Set the rollers slightly away from your scalp to "lift" your hair even more, combating the heavy look and feel you can get as layers grow out.
- Experiment with gels and barrettes and twisting to vary your look and help control the layers as they grow out.

GROWING OUT BANGS

Bangs should be trimmed regularly to keep them in shape and keep the ends from splitting during the growing-out process. Once they get to eyelash level, however, they can be very annoying. To lift them away from your eyes:

- Try setting them on a hot roller. Don't roll the roller tightly and secure it, however, or you'll end up with a "horn." Use one large roller and hold it with your fingers for a few seconds for a bit of lift and curve.
- Gather bangs with some side hair and twist the bangs and side hair into one section, which you can secure off your face with a comb, barrette, or headband.
- Try using gels and hair sprays to control stray hairs.

GROWING OUT A PERM

There are two major reasons for growing out a perm. One, you simply change your mind and want smooth, straight hair again or, two, the perm was improperly done and has damaged your hair. If you have changed your mind and your hair is in good condition, there are ways to relax a perm—check with your hairdresser.

Tips:

- To perk up a drooping perm that you are growing out, use hot rollers or get a spot perm of two or three strategically placed rods to give you a little bounce where needed.
- To improve damaged hair or if you decide to grow out the perm and skip the relaxing process, get frequent trims. You might also consider a very short style or a layered look to help remove as much of the perm as possible.
- Try controlling hair with combs and barrettes. You're at an advantage here because perming makes hair porous and the ornaments will "grip" and hold easily.

GROWING OUT COLOR

As with growing out a permanent, there are two reasons for growing out color: You have changed your mind, or the color was improperly done and has abused your hair.

Tips:

- If your hair is in good condition and you simply want to return to your natural color, consider reverse weaving, where a color matching your natural shade is laced into the colored hair to make the growing-out process less obvious.
- Try a wash-in haircolor that matches your natural shade.
- Consider layering hair or cutting it to a shorter length, especially if your hair has been damaged.

15 CREATING YOUR OWN HOME HAIR-GROOMING CENTER

You can have a workable, professional hair salon—tailor-made just for you—right in your own home. To create one all you need to have is the basic equipment required for the hairstyle you select and a place to organize and store it so that it's readily available for your use.

WHAT YOU NEED

Look at the chart for the hairstyle you have selected and gather the equipment listed under the heading "Tools and Appliances Required." Next, compile your shampoos, conditioners, and other hair-care products—refer to Chapter 13 for a guide to help you select them. Last, collect any hair ornaments you may want to use to vary your look.

Now is the perfect time to see what condition your equipment is in and decide what you need to buy to replace or supplement what you already own. Empty your bathroom, medicine cabinet, dressing table, drawers, and handbag of all your equipment and products and gather your finds in a big pile. Check each item to see if it is in proper condition. Review the discussions of tools and hair-care products in Chapters 8 and 13 before you go out and purchase whatever needs to be updated or added.

SETTING UP

For most women, the best and most practical place to locate your hair-grooming center is in your bathroom, where you'll be washing and treating your hair and working it—drying it, curling it, finishing it.

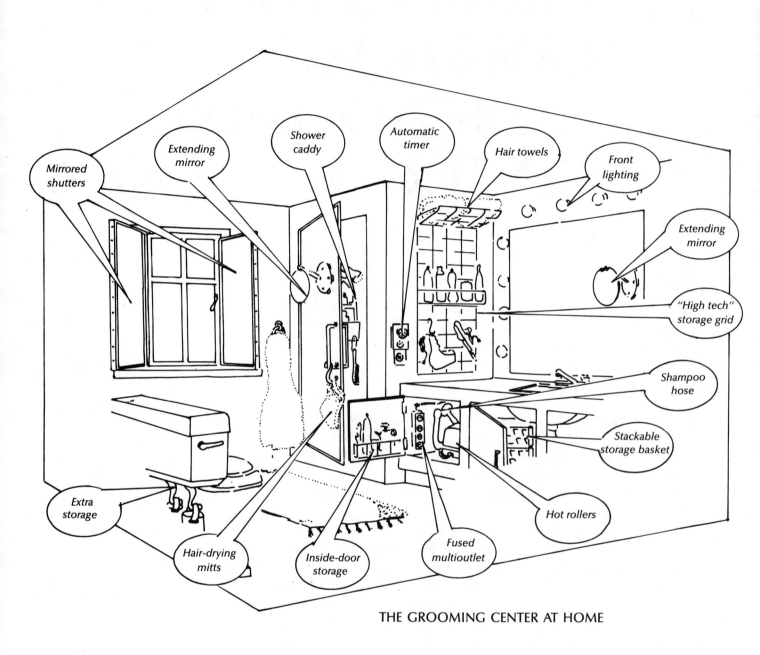

Mirrored shutters

Extending mirror

Shower caddy

Automatic timer

Hair towels

Front lighting

Extending mirror

"High tech" storage grid

Shampoo hose

Stackable storage basket

Extra storage

Hair-drying mitts

Inside-door storage

Fused multioutlet

Hot rollers

THE GROOMING CENTER AT HOME

Assess your bathroom's features. Do you have any drawers, counter area, shelves? Where are the electrical outlets? Your mirror? How is the lighting? If your bathroom doesn't have any area for storing equipment, buy and hang a set of shelves. If you have only one electrical outlet, get a three-way plug. If your mirror is small or inconveniently placed, install an extending mirror to provide back views of your head. Or try an auxiliary mirror that you can store in a drawer and hang on a window to give you direct light that shines right into your face. Still another idea is to cover the window with swing-out mirrored shutters.

You're also going to need good lighting, not merely an overhead light that you block out the moment you raise your hand to put in a roller. If necessary, install extra lights—an inexpensive clamp-on model might be the simplest approach—where needed.

TIPS FOR STORAGE

Store appliances out of the way by hanging them on hooks—screw-in cup hooks, glue-on plastic hooks, attractive brass or ceramic hooks. Assemble the hooks on the ceiling, under a windowsill, beneath the vanity, under a board attached to overhang the top of the toilet bowl, or on a mesh grid (the kind used for pots and pans). Use one hook for the appliance itself (if it doesn't have a ring with which to hang it, you can make one with a pretty ribbon). Use another hook for the cord (gather it up and secure it with a garbage bag twister).

● Keep bobby pins and hot roller pins handy by sticking them into a ball of modeling clay, Styrofoam, a stereo cleaner, a pop-up paper clip holder, around the edges of a mug (preferably not of glass), or on a magnet—you might want to attach the magnet to a wristband so you will have the pins right where you'll need them as you work on your hair. Hot roller pins store easily on empty thread spools, too, and you can color-code them to keep sizes separate and easy to recognize.

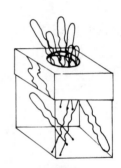

KEEP BOBBY PINS IN
A PAPER CLIP HOLDER . . .

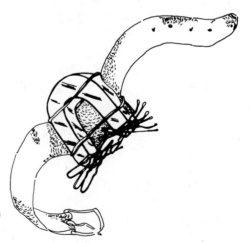

OR ON A MAGNET ATTACHED
TO A WRISTBAND

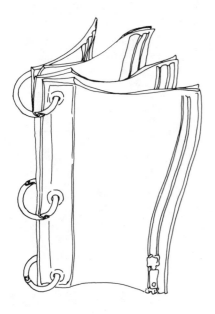

STORE CLIPS AND SPONGE
ROLLERS IN PLASTIC
PENCIL BAGS

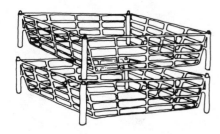

STACKABLE PLASTIC VEGETABLE
BINS ARE GOOD SPACE SAVERS

- Store clips, sponge rollers, and brushes in empty coffee cans you have painted or covered with fabric or wallpaper to match your bathroom decor, or in see-through jars that let you know at a glance what's inside and if you are running low on supplies. Or try plastic pencil bags—they are especially good for women who travel a lot because you can slip them right into a suitcase.
- Another clever way to store brushes: Clip them into a broom rack that's attached to a wall or behind the bathroom door.
- Collect covered bands around your mist bottle so you'll have them handy as you work.
- Use a shower caddy for shampoos, conditioners, and a wide-tooth comb tied to a rope, just like soap-on-a-rope.
- Use a tray with dividers or a silverware tray to separate and hold your collection of smaller items.
- To be decorative and inventive: Store items in old jam jars, antique porcelain boxes, sleek Lucite containers, rustic wicker baskets—any collection that suits your style.
- Gather your collection of boxes, jars, and bags on a tray so you can lift and place everything you need wherever you might be working.
- Store the tray in a drawer, on a counter, on a shelf, or in a stackable plastic vegetable bin under the basin or in a corner.
- One time-saving idea: Attach a timer to hot rollers or your curling iron so they can start heating up as you're waking up in the morning.

You may find that even with these space-maximizing ideas, you're short on space. In that case, you might want to divide your hair-grooming center into various working areas—the bathroom for "wet work" (where you'll need shampoos, conditioners, a wide-tooth comb); your bedroom or any area you find most convenient for "dry work" (station your dryer, a brush, and comb here); and a place for "finishing work" (where you'll need rollers, a curling iron, mist bottle, bobby pins, hairdressings, and ornaments).

Wherever you are working, you'll need plenty of elbowroom, mirror visibility, and good lighting.

The last item you'll want to have to complete your hair-grooming center: a book stand, so you can prop up a copy of this book to consult for your perfect hairstyle!

SAFETY COUNTS

It's a wise idea to make sure all your hair-care equipment and products are in good working order and stored properly. Here's a checklist of the major safety precautions:

✓ Check to see there are no tangles, kinks, or frays in cords of electrical appliances.

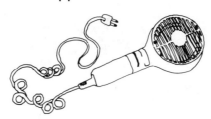

BE SURE TO UNTANGLE CORDS
OF ELECTRICAL APPLIANCES

✓ If you use a curling iron, look for one with a safety tip, and make sure the iron doesn't roll when you put it down. Keep curling irons away from children—they can mistake the rod for a handle.

✓ Make sure all hot appliances are cool—and unplugged—before children get near them. Remember to unplug appliances to avoid any chance of injury.

✓ Keep hair coloring out of the way—especially if you use powder packets, which can look like colored sugar to small children.

✓ If you use an extension cord, be sure that you work in a clear space so the cord doesn't catch on perfume bottles.

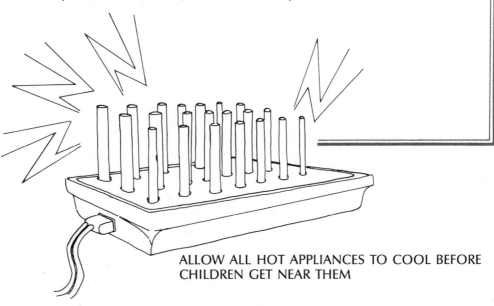

ALLOW ALL HOT APPLIANCES TO COOL BEFORE
CHILDREN GET NEAR THEM

16 DISCOVERING THE PERFECT HAIRSTYLE FOR *YOU*

Following are forty different hairstyle charts from which to choose your perfect style. These represent the very best looks in contemporary styling, from very short hair to very long, from simple and classic to sophisticated and breathtaking. There are hairstyles for day, evening, and every possible kind of look you might like to try. Study the photographs for each hairstyle and find the one or ones you like the best.

HOW TO USE THE CHARTS

1. Once you've found a hairstyle you'd like to try, go to the column on the chart called "Hair Type" and locate yours (numbers 1 to 27). To the right of your hair type you'll find a column labeled "Code." The Code tells you whether this is a good style for your hair. If you see that the style has a ■ code beside your hair type, the style is a *good* bet for you to try. If there is a □ code beside your hair type, the style is *possible* for you to try, but it may take some extra time for you to create. If the code next to your hair type is **X,** this means the style is not recommended for your hair, and you should keep looking through the charts.

You may discover a further notation in the Code column for the hairstyle you want to try. For example, let's say your hair type is number 11—medium texture, straight, medium quantity—and you see that the code for hair type number 11 on the chart is WP 14 ■. You know that the ■ means that this is a good style for you to try. The letters WP before the solid square stand for Wavy Perm, and they mean that before you can get the hairstyle pictured, you're going to have to change your hair's formation by getting a wavy perm. The number 14 is the hair type *you will become* after you have the wavy perm you need for the style. So, if your natural hair type is number 11 and you get the wavy perm you need for the hairstyle pictured, your hair type becomes number 14—medium texture, wavy, medium quantity. You've just improved your hair type (by bringing it closer to the mid-range of hair types) and expanded your hairstyling options. And you can now look through the charts and try the hairstyles you like that suit hair type 14.

Let's take another example. Suppose your hair type is number 4—fine texture, wavy, and thin. On the chart you see that the code for your hair type is C 13 ■. Again, the solid square indicates that this is a good style for you to attempt. The C stands for Coloring, and it tells you that to achieve this hairstyle, you need to change your hair's texture by adding some color. When you do, you become hair type 13—medium texture, wavy, and thin. Once again you've improved your natural hair type by getting closer to the desired midrange of types and have expanded the number of hairstyles to which your hair is suited. You're now ready to go through the hairstyle charts and select the styles you like to which hair type 13 is best suited.

The Code column indicates four types of changes you may have to make in order to achieve the style shown: S for Straightening, C for Coloring, WP for Wavy Perm, and CP for Curly Perm. Before you make any of these changes, you may want to review Chapter 5 for a discussion of what straightening, coloring, and perming can do for your hair.

2. When you've found a hairstyle you like and have determined by looking at the code for your hair type that it's a good style for you to try, you're ready to consider the time it will take, the skill rating you need, and the specific instructions for washing, setting, drying, and styling included on each of the charts. Read this information carefully. Be sure, too, to read the style hints for which facial features each style hides and highlights, the recommendations for body proportions, whether the style is Minimum Care or Temporary, and the tools and appliances required.

3. Finally, don't forget the Cutting Guide on each chart! This tells you exactly how your hair needs to be cut for the style and is an invaluable aid to you and your hairdresser. Be sure to show the

haircutting sketches and the photograph of the style you select to your hairdresser *before* he or she cuts your hair.

Reading the charts carefully is the best way to be certain you'll get the hairstyle you want exactly as it's pictured. It's as easy as that!

Congratulations—you've found your perfect hairstyle! We can't wait to see the beautiful new you!

THE
CHADWICK
HAIRSTYLES

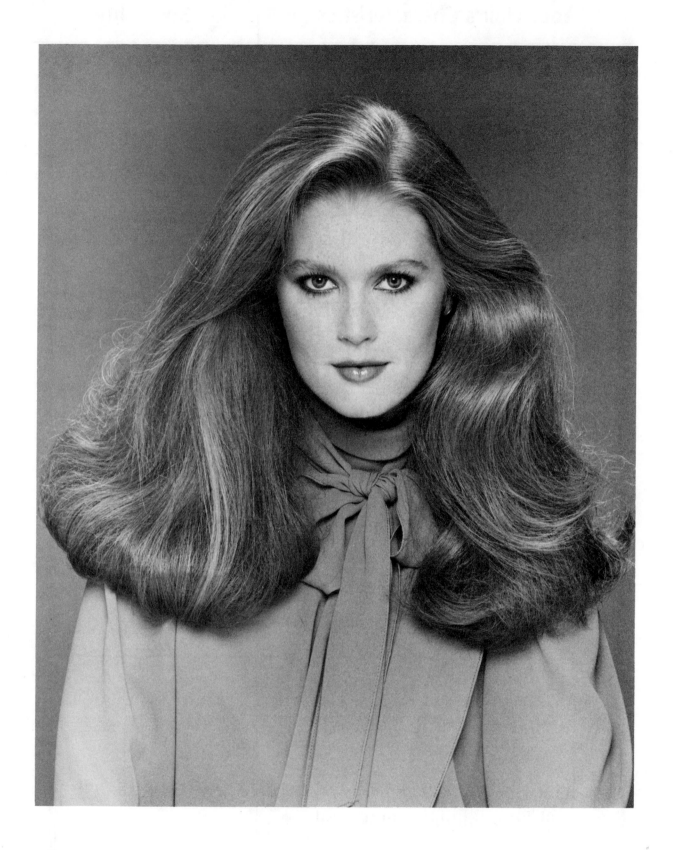

1 Controlled wave
for a smooth look

Your Hair's Characteristics | Stylability

TEXTURE	FORMATION	QUANTITY	HAIR TYPE	CODE	TIMING*	SKILL RATING
FINE	STRAIGHT	THIN	1	C10 ☐	30 to 45 mins.	3 to 4
		MEDIUM	2	C11 ☐		
		THICK	3	C12 ☐		
	WAVY	THIN	4	C13 ☐		
		MEDIUM	5	■		
		THICK	6	■		
	CURLY	THIN	7	X		
		MEDIUM	8	X		
		THICK	9	X		
MEDIUM	STRAIGHT	THIN	10	C19 ☐	30 to 45 mins.	3 to 4
		MEDIUM	11	C20 ☐		
		THICK	12	C21 ☐		
	WAVY	THIN	13	C22 ☐		
		MEDIUM	14	■		
		THICK	15	■		
	CURLY	THIN	16	X		
		MEDIUM	17	X		
		THICK	18	X		
COARSE	STRAIGHT	THIN	19	C20 ☐	30 to 45 mins.	3 to 4
		MEDIUM	20	C21 ☐		
		THICK	21	☐		
	WAVY	THIN	22	X		
		MEDIUM	23	■		
		THICK	24	■		
	CURLY	THIN	25	X		
		MEDIUM	26	X		
		THICK	27	X		

■ GOOD ☐ POSSIBLE X NOT RECOMMENDED

S STRAIGHTENING **C** COLORING **WP** WAVY PERM **CP** CURLY PERM

*25% extra time for porous hair

Finishing and Styling Hints

SPECIAL TIPS

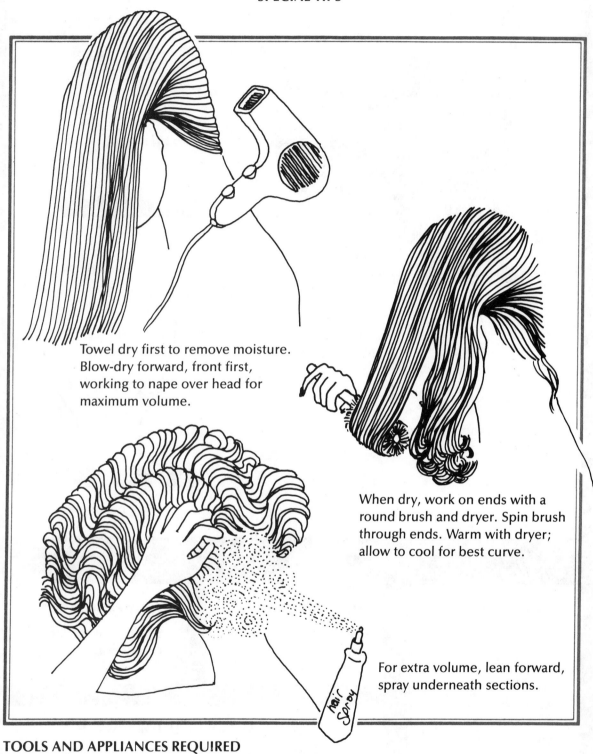

Towel dry first to remove moisture. Blow-dry forward, front first, working to nape over head for maximum volume.

When dry, work on ends with a round brush and dryer. Spin brush through ends. Warm with dryer; allow to cool for best curve.

For extra volume, lean forward, spray underneath sections.

TOOLS AND APPLIANCES REQUIRED

Towel
Wide-tooth Comb   Large-diameter round brush
Blow-dryer   Antistatic material (for fine textures)
Long clips   Hair spray (optional)

CUTTING GUIDE

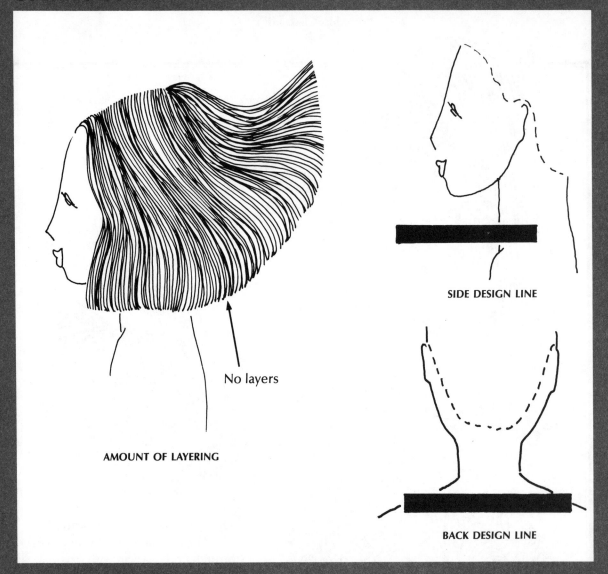

AMOUNT OF LAYERING

No layers

SIDE DESIGN LINE

BACK DESIGN LINE

THIS STYLE HIDES

Head size
Profile
Wide face
Chin
Jawline
Neck shapes: wide,
 short, thin, long

THIS STYLE HIGHLIGHTS

Hair condition
Long face
Front hairline

BODY PROPORTIONS

Suitable for medium-to-
tall proportions

THIS IS A *MINIMUM CARE* STYLE FOR WAVY HAIR.

THIS IS A *TEMPORARY* STYLE FOR STRAIGHT HAIR.

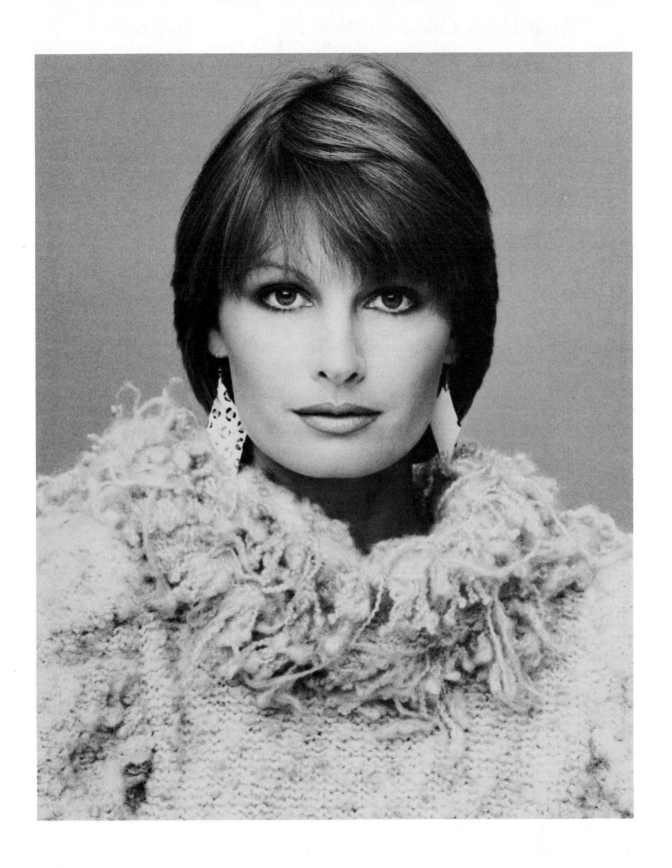

2 Neat and soft

Your Hair's Characteristics | Stylability

TEXTURE	FORMATION	QUANTITY	HAIR TYPE	CODE	TIMING*	SKILL RATING
FINE	STRAIGHT	THIN	1	C10 ■	15 to 20 mins.	1 to 3
FINE	STRAIGHT	MEDIUM	2	■		
FINE	STRAIGHT	THICK	3	■		
FINE	WAVY	THIN	4	C13 □		
FINE	WAVY	MEDIUM	5	□		
FINE	WAVY	THICK	6	□		
FINE	CURLY	THIN	7	X		
FINE	CURLY	MEDIUM	8	X		
FINE	CURLY	THICK	9	S3 □		
MEDIUM	STRAIGHT	THIN	10	C19 ■	15 to 20 mins.	1 to 3
MEDIUM	STRAIGHT	MEDIUM	11	■		
MEDIUM	STRAIGHT	THICK	12	■		
MEDIUM	WAVY	THIN	13	C22 □		
MEDIUM	WAVY	MEDIUM	14	□		
MEDIUM	WAVY	THICK	15	□		
MEDIUM	CURLY	THIN	16	S10 ■		
MEDIUM	CURLY	MEDIUM	17	S11 ■		
MEDIUM	CURLY	THICK	18	S12 ■		
COARSE	STRAIGHT	THIN	19	C20 ■	15 to 20 mins.	1 to 3
COARSE	STRAIGHT	MEDIUM	20	■		
COARSE	STRAIGHT	THICK	21	■		
COARSE	WAVY	THIN	22	C23 □		
COARSE	WAVY	MEDIUM	23	□		
COARSE	WAVY	THICK	24	□		
COARSE	CURLY	THIN	25	S19 ■		
COARSE	CURLY	MEDIUM	26	S20 ■		
COARSE	CURLY	THICK	27	S21 ■		

96

■ GOOD   □ POSSIBLE   X NOT RECOMMENDED

S STRAIGHTENING   C COLORING   WP WAVY PERM   CP CURLY PERM

*25% extra time for porous hair

Finishing and Styling Hints

SPECIAL TIPS

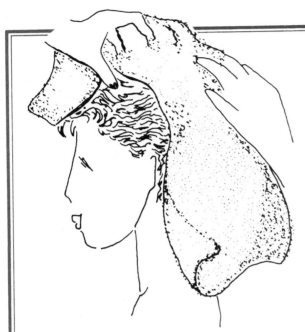

Towel dry to remove excess moisture.

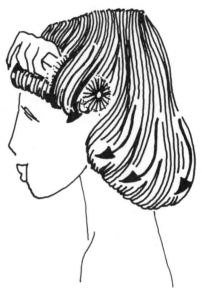

On wavy hair, after towel drying, spin a large-diameter brush through ends. Apply blow-dryer; warm hair until all ends turn under. Brush away from face and sides with a vent or Denman brush; shake into position.

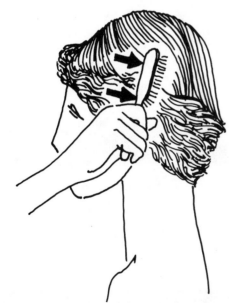

On straight hair, part for style and, with a vent or Denman brush and blow-dryer, brush and dry hair away from face and away from sides leading down into nape.

TOOLS AND APPLIANCES REQUIRED

Towel
Wide-tooth comb
Denman or vent brush
Blow-dryer
Large-diameter round brush

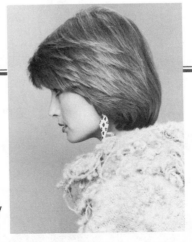

SIDE VIEW

CUTTING GUIDE

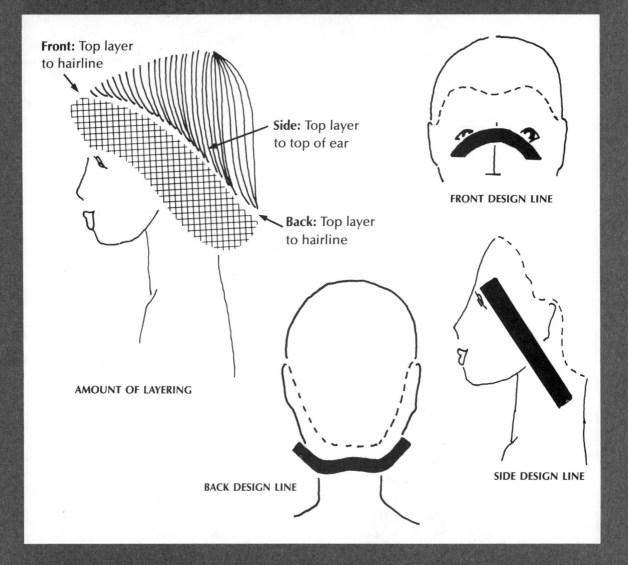

Front: Top layer to hairline

Side: Top layer to top of ear

Back: Top layer to hairline

AMOUNT OF LAYERING

FRONT DESIGN LINE

BACK DESIGN LINE

SIDE DESIGN LINE

THIS STYLE HIDES

Ears
All hairlines
Large forehead
Wide or narrow temples
Sparse hair at temples
Profile
Head shape

THIS STYLE HIGHLIGHTS

Hair condition
Head size
Chin
Jawline

BODY PROPORTIONS

Not suitable for large proportions

THIS IS A *MINIMUM CARE* STYLE FOR STRAIGHT HAIR.

THIS IS A *TEMPORARY* STYLE FOR WAVY HAIR.

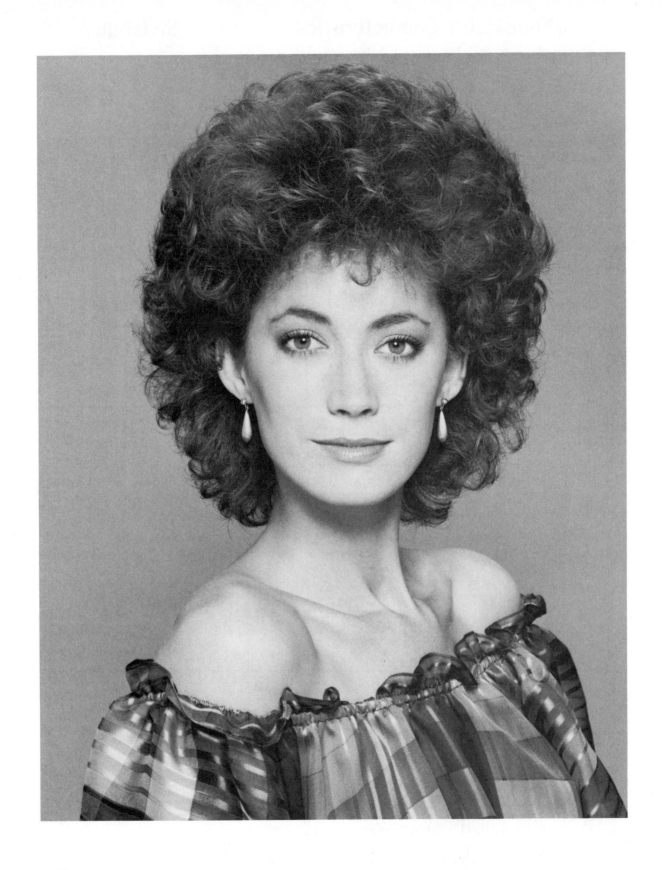

3 The full, natural look for curly hair

TEXTURE	FORMATION		QUANTITY	HAIR TYPE	CODE	TIMING*	SKILL RATING
FINE	STRAIGHT		THIN	1	CP7 ■		
			MEDIUM	2	CP8 ■		
			THICK	3	CP9 ■		
	WAVY		THIN	4	CP13 □	20 to 30 mins.	2 to 3
			MEDIUM	5	□		
			THICK	6	□		
	CURLY		THIN	7	C16 ■		
			MEDIUM	8	■		
			THICK	9	■		
MEDIUM	STRAIGHT		THIN	10	CP16 ■		
			MEDIUM	11	CP17 ■		
			THICK	12	CP18 ■		
	WAVY		THIN	13	C22 □	20 to 30 mins.	2 to 3
			MEDIUM	14	□		
			THICK	15	□		
	CURLY		THIN	16	■		
			MEDIUM	17	■		
			THICK	18	■		
COARSE	STRAIGHT		THIN	19	CP25 ■		
			MEDIUM	20	CP26 ■		
			THICK	21	CP27 ■		
	WAVY		THIN	22	C23 □	20 to 30 mins.	2 to 3
			MEDIUM	23	□		
			THICK	24	□		
	CURLY		THIN	25	■		
			MEDIUM	26	■		
			THICK	27	■		

100

■ GOOD   □ POSSIBLE   X NOT RECOMMENDED   S STRAIGHTENING   C COLORING   WP WAVY PERM   CP CURLY PERM

*25% extra time for porous hair

Finishing and Styling Hints

SPECIAL TIPS

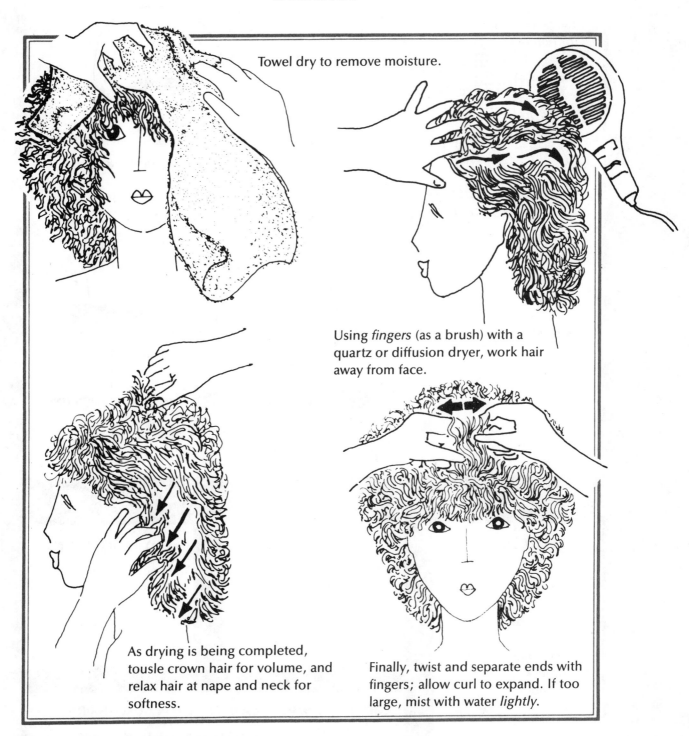

Towel dry to remove moisture.

Using *fingers* (as a brush) with a quartz or diffusion dryer, work hair away from face.

As drying is being completed, tousle crown hair for volume, and relax hair at nape and neck for softness.

Finally, twist and separate ends with fingers; allow curl to expand. If too large, mist with water *lightly*.

TOOLS AND APPLIANCES REQUIRED

Towel
Wide-tooth comb
Quartz or diffusion dryer
Mist Bottle
Hair spray (optional)
Spray shine (optional)

CUTTING GUIDE

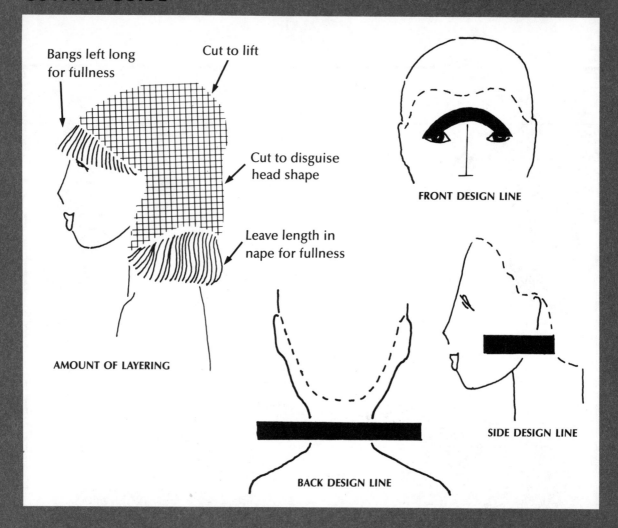

Bangs left long for fullness

Cut to lift

Cut to disguise head shape

Leave length in nape for fullness

AMOUNT OF LAYERING

FRONT DESIGN LINE

SIDE DESIGN LINE

BACK DESIGN LINE

THIS STYLE HIDES

Head shape
Head size
Profile
Low forehead
Front hairline
Nape hairline
Short neck
Hair condition

THIS STYLE HIGHLIGHTS

Ears
Face shape
Chin
Jawline
Hairline in front of ears

BODY PROPORTIONS

Suitable for medium, tall, and large proportions

THIS IS A *MINIMUM CARE* STYLE FOR CURLY HAIR.

THIS IS A *TEMPORARY* STYLE FOR STRAIGHT HAIR.

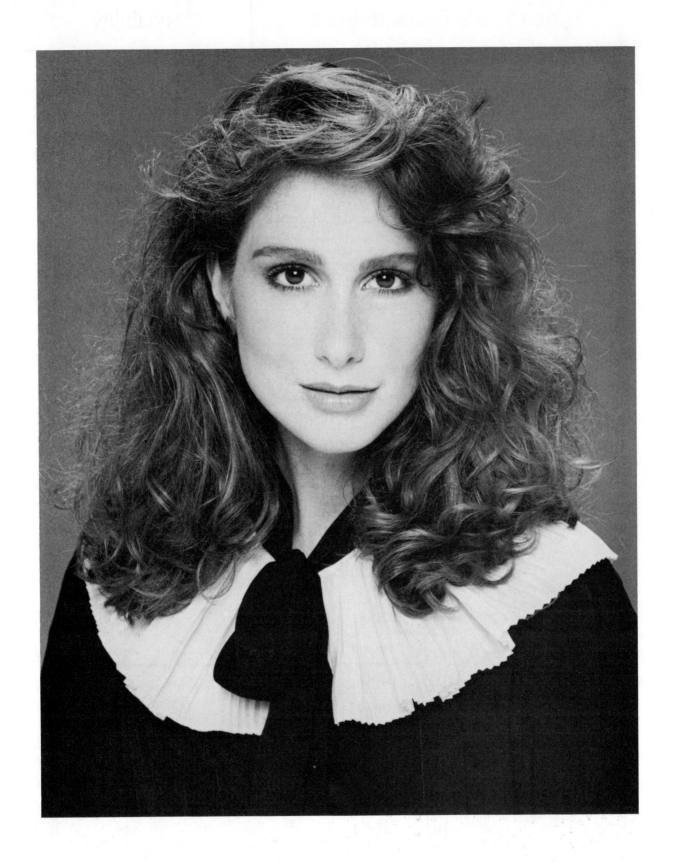

4 Lightly layered

Your Hair's Characteristics | Stylability

TEXTURE	FORMATION	QUANTITY	HAIR TYPE	CODE	TIMING*	SKILL RATING
FINE	STRAIGHT	THIN	1	WP4 ■	20 to 35 mins.	2 to 3
FINE	STRAIGHT	MEDIUM	2	WP5 ■		
FINE	STRAIGHT	THICK	3	WP6 ■		
FINE	WAVY	THIN	4	C13 ■		
FINE	WAVY	MEDIUM	5	■		
FINE	WAVY	THICK	6	■		
FINE	CURLY	THIN	7	X		
FINE	CURLY	MEDIUM	8	X		
FINE	CURLY	THICK	9	X		
MEDIUM	STRAIGHT	THIN	10	WP13 ■	20 to 35 mins.	2 to 3
MEDIUM	STRAIGHT	MEDIUM	11	WP14 ■		
MEDIUM	STRAIGHT	THICK	12	WP15 ■		
MEDIUM	WAVY	THIN	13	C22 ■		
MEDIUM	WAVY	MEDIUM	14	■		
MEDIUM	WAVY	THICK	15	■		
MEDIUM	CURLY	THIN	16	X		
MEDIUM	CURLY	MEDIUM	17	X		
MEDIUM	CURLY	THICK	18	X		
COARSE	STRAIGHT	THIN	19	WP22 ■	20 to 35 mins.	2 to 3
COARSE	STRAIGHT	MEDIUM	20	WP23 ■		
COARSE	STRAIGHT	THICK	21	WP24 ■		
COARSE	WAVY	THIN	22	■		
COARSE	WAVY	MEDIUM	23	■		
COARSE	WAVY	THICK	24	■		
COARSE	CURLY	THIN	25	X		
COARSE	CURLY	MEDIUM	26	X		
COARSE	CURLY	THICK	27	X		

■ GOOD   □ POSSIBLE   X NOT RECOMMENDED   S STRAIGHTENING   C COLORING   **WP** WAVY PERM   **CP** CURLY PERM

104

*25% extra time for porous hair

Finishing and Styling Hints

SPECIAL TIPS

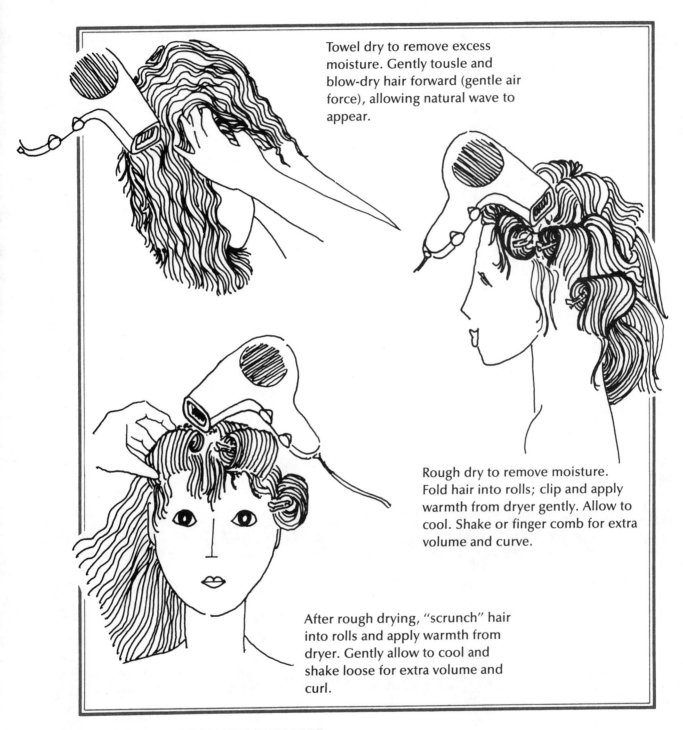

Towel dry to remove excess moisture. Gently tousle and blow-dry hair forward (gentle air force), allowing natural wave to appear.

Rough dry to remove moisture. Fold hair into rolls; clip and apply warmth from dryer gently. Allow to cool. Shake or finger comb for extra volume and curve.

After rough drying, "scrunch" hair into rolls and apply warmth from dryer. Gently allow to cool and shake loose for extra volume and curl.

TOOLS AND APPLIANCES REQUIRED
Towel
Wide-tooth comb
Blow-dryer (variable air power)
Short clips
Hair spray (optional)

CUTTING GUIDE

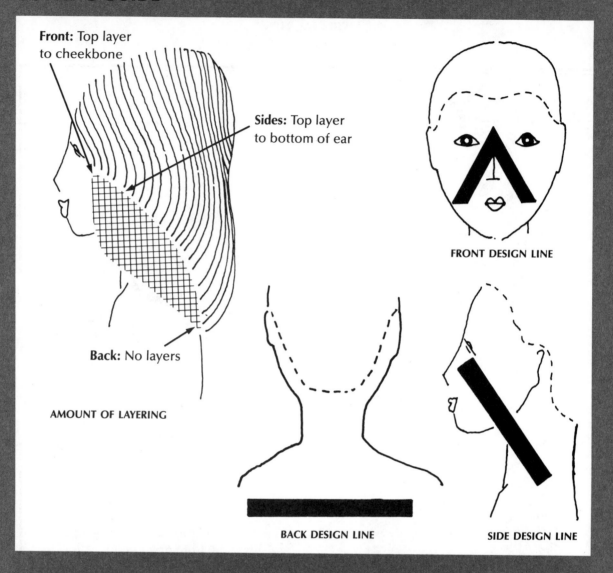

Front: Top layer to cheekbone

Sides: Top layer to bottom of ear

Back: No layers

AMOUNT OF LAYERING

FRONT DESIGN LINE

BACK DESIGN LINE

SIDE DESIGN LINE

THIS STYLE HIDES

Head shape
Head size
Profile
Ears
Face shape
Chin
Jawline
All hairlines
Neck shapes: wide,
   short, long, thin

THIS STYLE HIGHLIGHTS

Hair condition

BODY PROPORTIONS

Suitable for small,
medium, large, and
tall proportions

THIS IS A *MINIMUM CARE* STYLE FOR WAVY-TO-CURLY HAIR.

THIS IS A *TEMPORARY* STYLE FOR STRAIGHT HAIR.

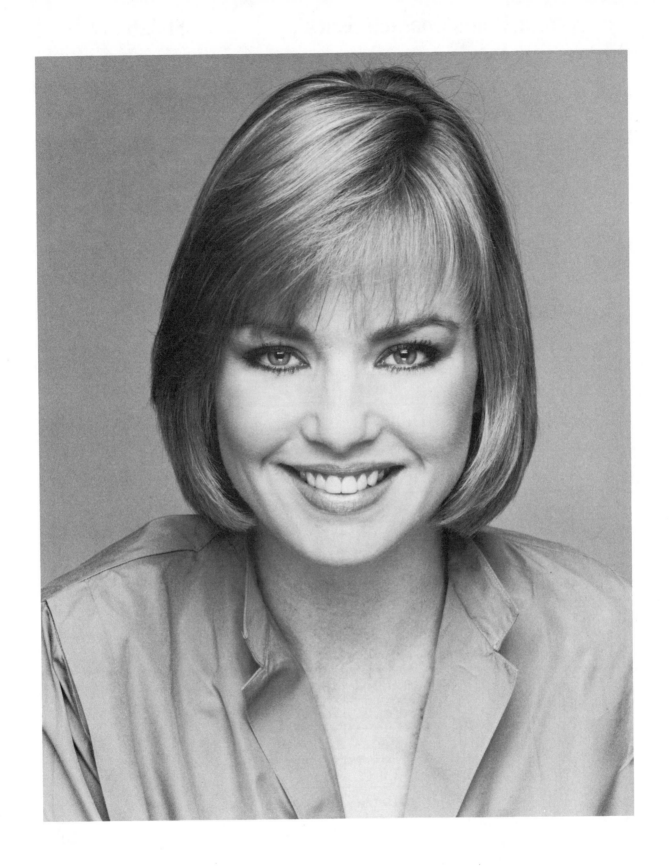

5 Wispy bob

TEXTURE	FORMATION	QUANTITY	HAIR TYPE	CODE	TIMING*	SKILL RATING
FINE	STRAIGHT	THIN	1	C10 ■	15 to 20 mins.	2 to 3
		MEDIUM	2	■		
		THICK	3	■		
	WAVY	THIN	4	C13 □		
		MEDIUM	5	□		
		THICK	6	□		
	CURLY	THIN	7	X		
		MEDIUM	8	X		
		THICK	9	■		
MEDIUM	STRAIGHT	THIN	10	■	15 to 20 mins.	2 to 3
		MEDIUM	11	■		
		THICK	12	■		
	WAVY	THIN	13	C22 □		
		MEDIUM	14	□		
		THICK	15	□		
	CURLY	THIN	16	S10 ■		
		MEDIUM	17	S11 ■		
		THICK	18	S12 ■		
COARSE	STRAIGHT	THIN	19	■	20 to 25 mins.	2 to 3
		MEDIUM	20	■		
		THICK	21	■		
	WAVY	THIN	22	C23 □		
		MEDIUM	23	C24 □		
		THICK	24	□		
	CURLY	THIN	25	S19 ■		
		MEDIUM	26	S20 ■		
		THICK	27	S21 ■		

■ GOOD   □ POSSIBLE   X NOT RECOMMENDED   S STRAIGHTENING   C COLORING   **WP** WAVY PERM   **CP** CURLY PERM

*25% extra time for porous hair

Finishing and Styling Hints

SPECIAL TIPS

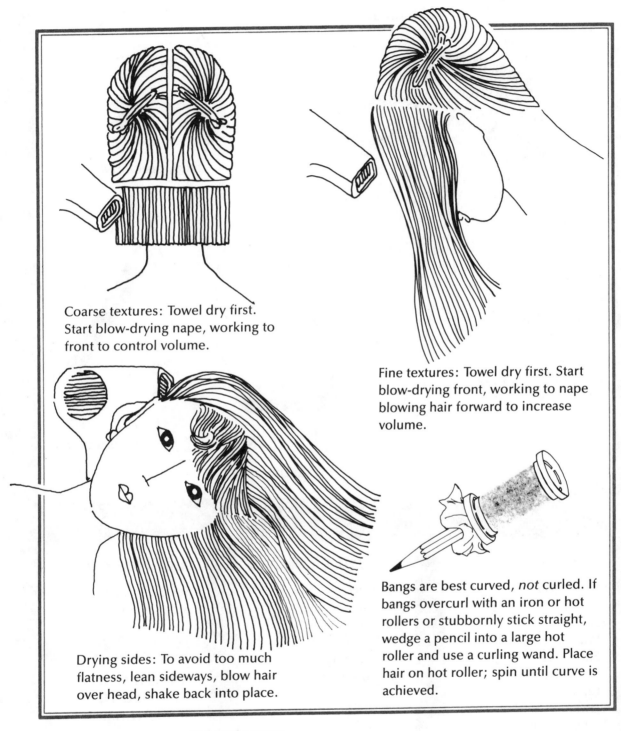

Coarse textures: Towel dry first. Start blow-drying nape, working to front to control volume.

Fine textures: Towel dry first. Start blow-drying front, working to nape blowing hair forward to increase volume.

Drying sides: To avoid too much flatness, lean sideways, blow hair over head, shake back into place.

Bangs are best curved, *not* curled. If bangs overcurl with an iron or hot rollers or stubbornly stick straight, wedge a pencil into a large hot roller and use a curling wand. Place hair on hot roller; spin until curve is achieved.

TOOLS AND APPLIANCES REQUIRED
Towel
Wide-tooth comb
Denman or vent brush
Blow-dryer
Long clips
Antistatic material (for fine textures)
Hot roller on a pencil (optional)

CUTTING GUIDE

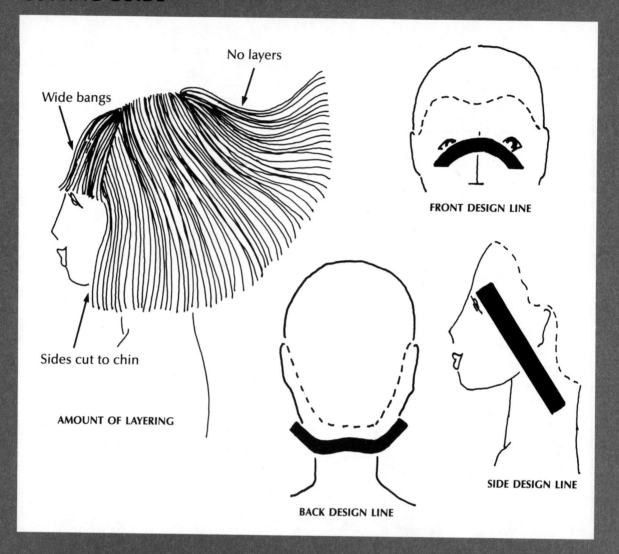

Wide bangs

No layers

Sides cut to chin

AMOUNT OF LAYERING

FRONT DESIGN LINE

BACK DESIGN LINE

SIDE DESIGN LINE

THIS STYLE HIDES

Head shape
Profile
Ears
Wide face
Short face
Chubby cheeks
Chin
Jawline
All hairlines

THIS STYLE HIGHLIGHTS

Head size
Thin face
Long face
Neck shapes: wide,
   short, long, thin
Hair condition

BODY PROPORTIONS

Suitable for all
proportions

THIS IS A *MINIMUM CARE* STYLE FOR STRAIGHT HAIR.

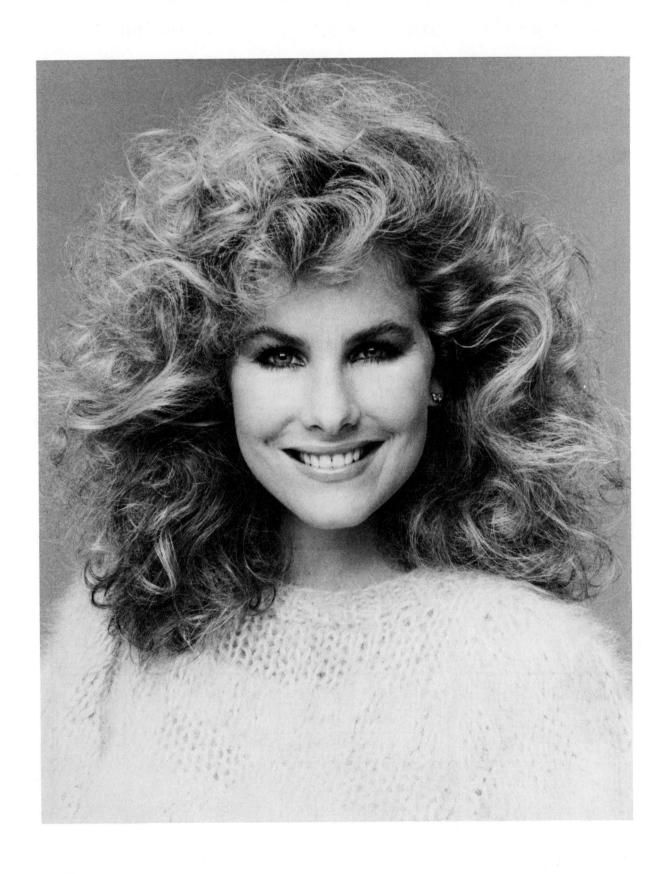

6 Curls galore

Your Hair's Characteristics / Stylability

TEXTURE	FORMATION	QUANTITY	HAIR TYPE	CODE	TIMING*	SKILL RATING
FINE	STRAIGHT	THIN	1	WP4 ☐	35 to 45 mins.	3 to 4
		MEDIUM	2	WP5 ☐		
		THICK	3	WP6 ☐		
	WAVY	THIN	4	C13 ☐		
		MEDIUM	5	☐		
		THICK	6	☐		
	CURLY	THIN	7	C16 ■		
		MEDIUM	8	■		
		THICK	9	■		
MEDIUM	STRAIGHT	THIN	10	CP16 ■	35 to 45 mins.	3 to 4
		MEDIUM	11	CP17 ■		
		THICK	12	CP18 ■		
	WAVY	THIN	13	C22 ☐		
		MEDIUM	14	☐		
		THICK	15	☐		
	CURLY	THIN	16	C25 ■		
		MEDIUM	17	■		
		THICK	18	■		
COARSE	STRAIGHT	THIN	19	WP22 ☐	35 to 50 mins.	3 to 4
		MEDIUM	20	WP23 ☐		
		THICK	21	WP24 ☐		
	WAVY	THIN	22	C23 ☐		
		MEDIUM	23	☐		
		THICK	24	☐		
	CURLY	THIN	25	C26 ■		
		MEDIUM	26	■		
		THICK	27	■		

■ GOOD ☐ POSSIBLE X NOT RECOMMENDED   S STRAIGHTENING C COLORING WP WAVY PERM CP CURLY PERM

*25% extra time for porous hair

Finishing and Styling Hints

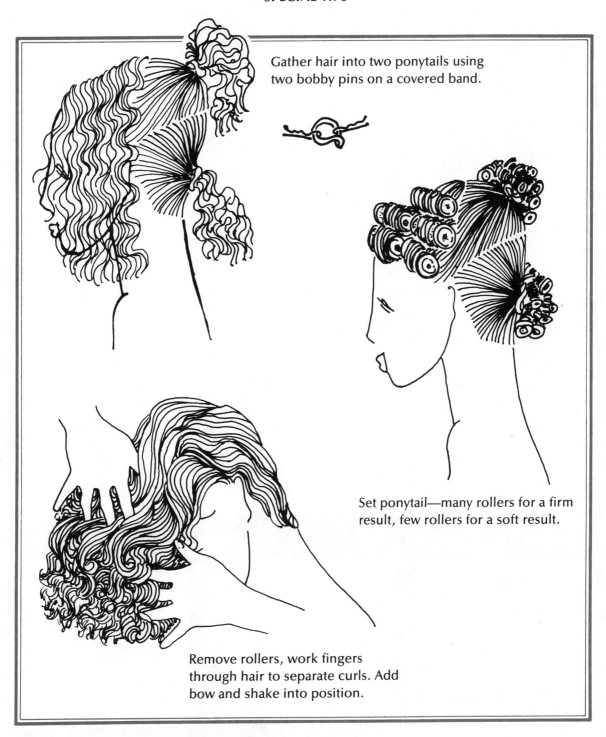

Gather hair into two ponytails using two bobby pins on a covered band.

Set ponytail—many rollers for a firm result, few rollers for a soft result.

Remove rollers, work fingers through hair to separate curls. Add bow and shake into position.

TOOLS AND APPLIANCES REQUIRED

Towel	Hot rollers
Wide-tooth comb	Covered bands with bobby pins
Rattail comb	Ribbon
Denman or vent brush	Hair spray (optional)
Blow-dryer	Antistatic material (for fine hair—optional)

CUTTING GUIDE

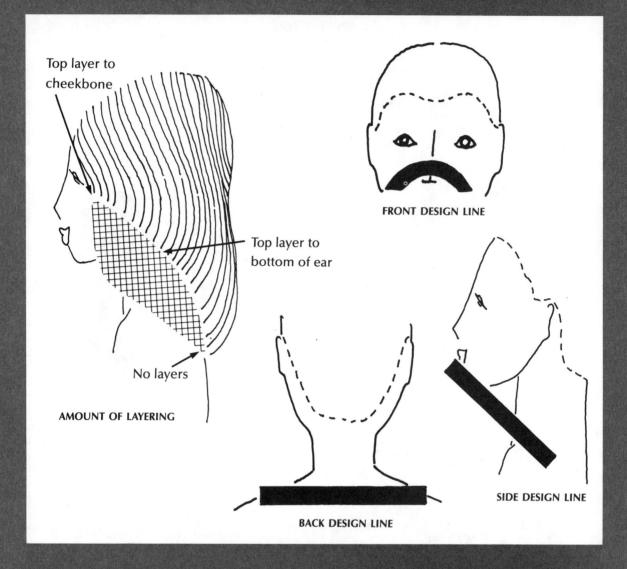

Top layer to cheekbone

Top layer to bottom of ear

No layers

AMOUNT OF LAYERING

FRONT DESIGN LINE

SIDE DESIGN LINE

BACK DESIGN LINE

THIS STYLE HIDES

Head shape
Head size
Profile
Ears
Face shape
Chubby cheeks
Chin
Jawline
Low forehead
Nape hairline
Hairline in front of ears
Neck shapes: wide,
    short, long, thin

THIS STYLE HIGHLIGHTS

Receding hairline
Narrow temples
Wide temples
Sparse hair at temples
Front hairline
Hair condition

BODY PROPORTIONS

Suitable for medium,
tall, and large
proportions

THIS IS A *MINIMUM CARE* STYLE FOR WAVY-TO-CURLY HAIR.

THIS IS A *TEMPORARY* STYLE FOR STRAIGHT HAIR.

114

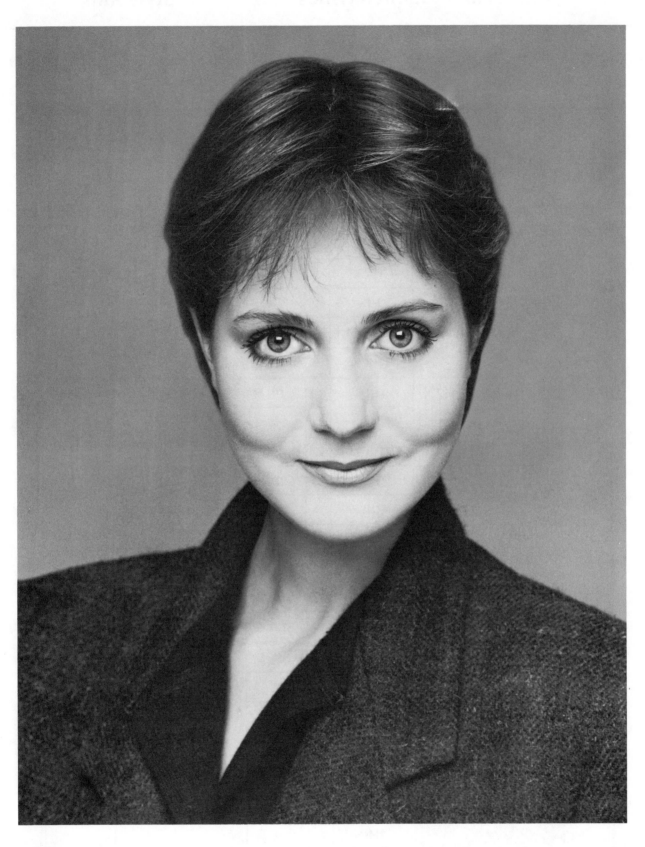

7 Simply cut for the chic, tailored look

Your Hair's Characteristics | Stylability

TEXTURE	FORMATION	QUANTITY	HAIR TYPE	CODE	TIMING*	SKILL RATING
FINE	STRAIGHT	THIN	1	C10 ■	10 to 20 mins.	2 to 3
		MEDIUM	2	■		
		THICK	3	■		
	WAVY	THIN	4	C13 □		
		MEDIUM	5	□		
		THICK	6	□		
	CURLY	THIN	7	X		
		MEDIUM	8	X		
		THICK	9	S3 ■		
MEDIUM	STRAIGHT	THIN	10	C19 ■	10 to 20 mins.	2 to 3
		MEDIUM	11	■		
		THICK	12	■		
	WAVY	THIN	13	C22 □		
		MEDIUM	14	□		
		THICK	15	□		
	CURLY	THIN	16	S10 ■		
		MEDIUM	17	S11 ■		
		THICK	18	S12 ■		
COARSE	STRAIGHT	THIN	19	C 20 ■	10 to 20 mins.	2 to 3
		MEDIUM	20	■		
		THICK	21	■		
	WAVY	THIN	22	C23 □		
		MEDIUM	23	□		
		THICK	24	□		
	CURLY	THIN	25	S19 ■		
		MEDIUM	26	S20 ■		
		THICK	27	S21 ■		

■ GOOD □ POSSIBLE X NOT RECOMMENDED S STRAIGHTENING C COLORING WP WAVY PERM CP CURLY PERM

*25% extra time for porous hair

Finishing and Styling Hints

SPECIAL TIPS

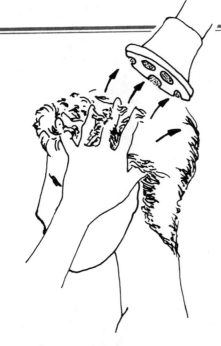

For curly hair: Towel dry first. Using fingers and a diffusion dryer, work hair off face. Allow curl to form style.

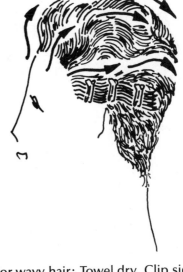

For wavy hair: Towel dry. Clip sides, and with a Denman or vent brush, blow-dry from front to back.

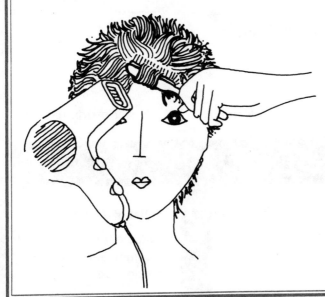

For straight hair: Towel dry. With a Denman or vent brush, blow-dry off face to crown. **Note:** For extra curve, lock hair into brush, apply warm air to section, and flip into shape.

TOOLS AND APPLIANCES REQUIRED
Towel
Vent and/or Denman brush
Blow-dryer
Diffusion dryer
Short clips

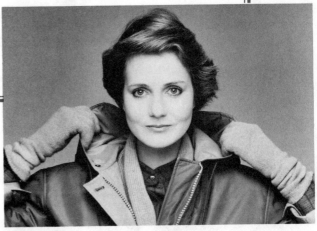

VARIATION

CUTTING GUIDE

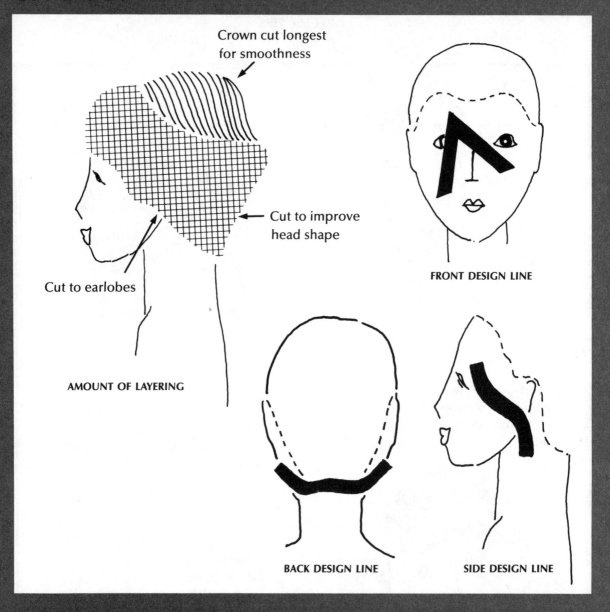

Crown cut longest for smoothness

Cut to improve head shape

Cut to earlobes

AMOUNT OF LAYERING

FRONT DESIGN LINE

BACK DESIGN LINE

SIDE DESIGN LINE

THIS STYLE HIDES

Head shape
Profile
Short face
Receding hairline
Low forehead
Narrow temples
Sparse hair at temples
Wide temples
Front hairline
Nape hairline

THIS STYLE HIGHLIGHTS

Head size
Ears
Face shape
Chin
Jawline
Hairline in front of ears
Neck shapes: wide,
   short, long, thin
Hair condition

BODY PROPORTIONS

Suitable for petite, small, medium, and tall proportions

THIS IS A *MINIMUM CARE* STYLE FOR STRAIGHT-TO-WAVY HAIR.

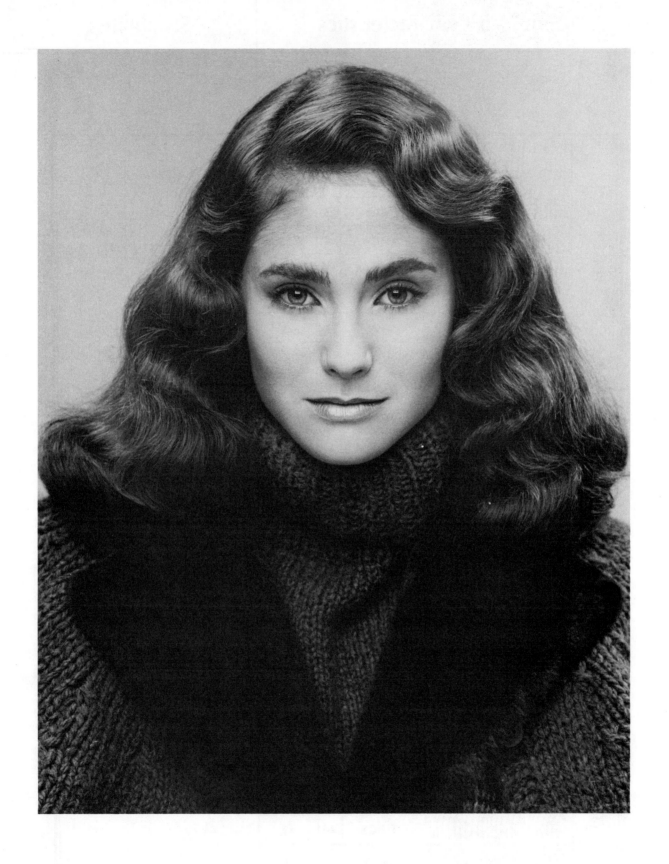

8 Waved bob

Your Hair's Characteristics — Stylability

TEXTURE	FORMATION	QUANTITY	HAIR TYPE	CODE	TIMING*	SKILL RATING
FINE	STRAIGHT	THIN	1	WP4 ■		
		MEDIUM	2	WP5 ■		
		THICK	3	WP6 ■		
	WAVY	THIN	4	C13 ■	40 to 50 mins.	3 to 4
		MEDIUM	5	■		
		THICK	6	■		
	CURLY	THIN	7	X		
		MEDIUM	8	X		
		THICK	9	X		
MEDIUM	STRAIGHT	THIN	10	WP13 ■		
		MEDIUM	11	WP14 ■		
		THICK	12	WP15 ■		
	WAVY	THIN	13	■	40 to 50 mins.	3 to 4
		MEDIUM	14	■		
		THICK	15	■		
	CURLY	THIN	16	X		
		MEDIUM	17	X		
		THICK	18	X		
COARSE	STRAIGHT	THIN	19	WP22 ■		
		MEDIUM	20	WP23 ■		
		THICK	21	WP24 ■		
	WAVY	THIN	22	■	40 to 50 mins.	3 to 4
		MEDIUM	23	■		
		THICK	24	■		
	CURLY	THIN	25	X		
		MEDIUM	26	X		
		THICK	27	X		

■ GOOD   □ POSSIBLE   X NOT RECOMMENDED

S STRAIGHTENING   C COLORING   WP WAVY PERM   CP CURLY PERM

*25% extra time for porous hair

Finishing and Styling Hints

SPECIAL TIPS

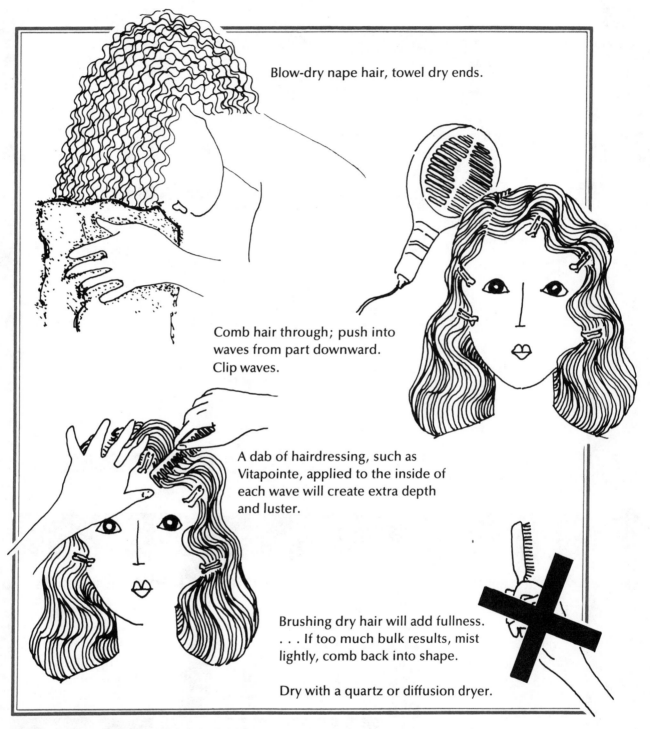

Blow-dry nape hair, towel dry ends.

Comb hair through; push into waves from part downward. Clip waves.

A dab of hairdressing, such as Vitapointe, applied to the inside of each wave will create extra depth and luster.

Brushing dry hair will add fullness. . . . If too much bulk results, mist lightly, comb back into shape.

Dry with a quartz or diffusion dryer.

TOOLS AND APPLIANCES REQUIRED
Towel
Blow-dryer
Wide-tooth comb
Short clips
Quartz or diffusion dryer
Hairdressing, such as Vitapointe, or spray shine (optional)

CUTTING GUIDE

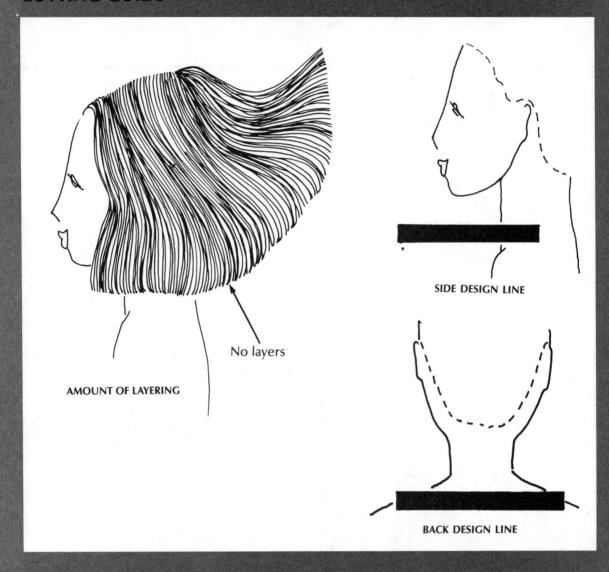

AMOUNT OF LAYERING

No layers

SIDE DESIGN LINE

BACK DESIGN LINE

THIS STYLE HIDES

Head shape
Head size
Profile
Ears
Face shape
Wide face
Chubby cheeks
Chin
Jawline
Nape hairline
Hairline in front of ears
Neck shapes: wide,
   short, long, or thin

THIS STYLE HIGHLIGHTS

Thin face
Long face
Receding hairline
Narrow temples
Front hairline
Hair condition

BODY PROPORTIONS

Suitable for medium, tall, and large proportions; should be *avoided* by petite and small proportions

THIS IS A *MINIMUM CARE* STYLE FOR WAVY-TO-CURLY HAIR.

THIS IS A *TEMPORARY* STYLE FOR STRAIGHT HAIR.

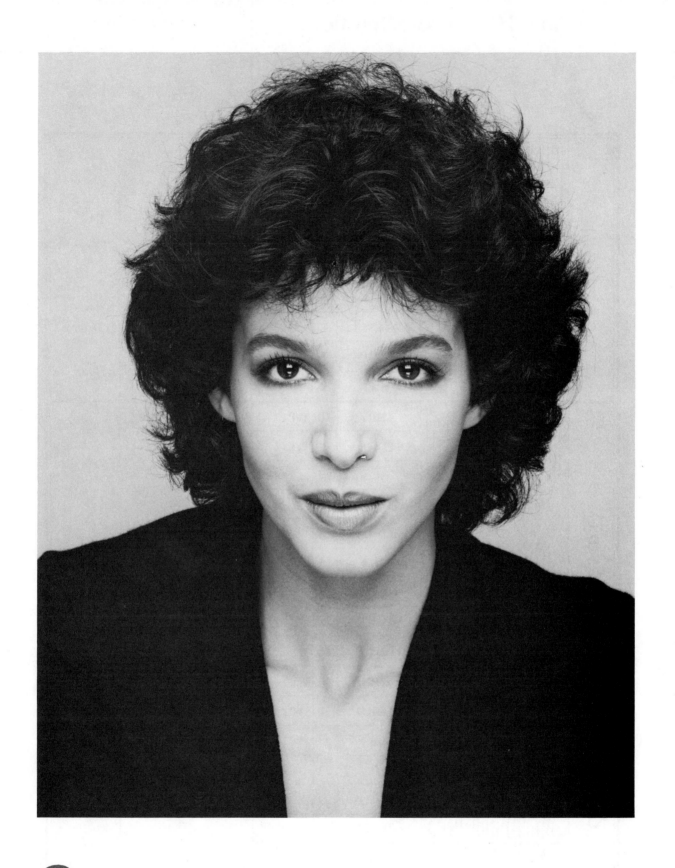

9 Practical and pretty for daytime

Your Hair's Characteristics | Stylability

TEXTURE	FORMATION	QUANTITY	HAIR TYPE	CODE	TIMING*	SKILL RATING
FINE	STRAIGHT	THIN	1	WP4 ■	10 to 15 mins.	2
		MEDIUM	2	WP5 ■		
		THICK	3	WP6 ■		
	WAVY	THIN	4	C13 ■		
		MEDIUM	5	■		
		THICK	6	■		
	CURLY	THIN	7	C16 ■		
		MEDIUM	8	■		
		THICK	9	■		
MEDIUM	STRAIGHT	THIN	10	WP13 ■	15 to 20 mins.	2
		MEDIUM	11	WP14 ■		
		THICK	12	WP15 ■		
	WAVY	THIN	13	C22 ■		
		MEDIUM	14	■		
		THICK	15	■		
	CURLY	THIN	16	C25 ■		
		MEDIUM	17	■		
		THICK	18	■		
COARSE	STRAIGHT	THIN	19	WP22 ■	20 to 25 mins.	3
		MEDIUM	20	WP23 ■		
		THICK	21	WP24 ■		
	WAVY	THIN	22	C23 ■		
		MEDIUM	23	■		
		THICK	24	■		
	CURLY	THIN	25	C26 ■		
		MEDIUM	26	■		
		THICK	27	■		

■ GOOD   ☐ POSSIBLE   X NOT RECOMMENDED

S STRAIGHTENING **C** COLORING **WP** WAVY PERM **CP** CURLY PERM

*25% extra time for porous hair

124

Finishing and Styling Hints

SPECIAL TIPS

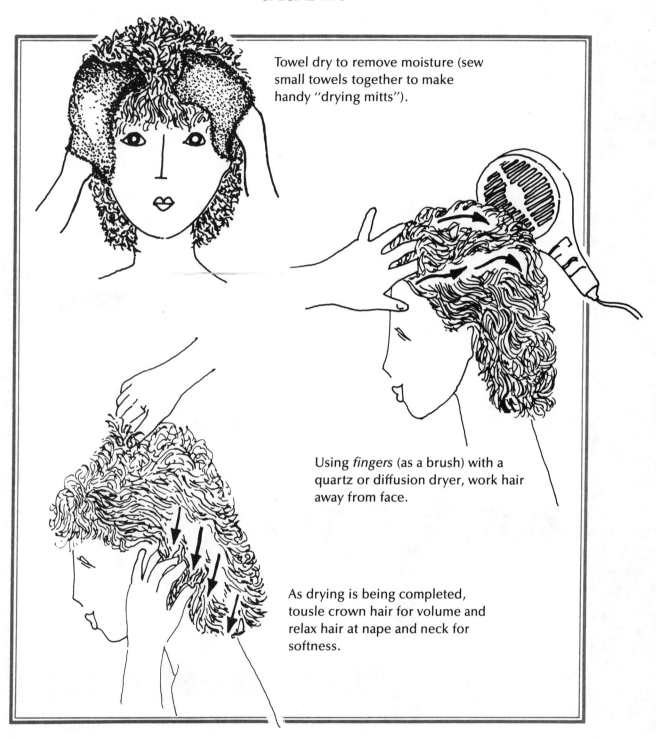

Towel dry to remove moisture (sew small towels together to make handy "drying mitts").

Using *fingers* (as a brush) with a quartz or diffusion dryer, work hair away from face.

As drying is being completed, tousle crown hair for volume and relax hair at nape and neck for softness.

TOOLS AND APPLIANCES REQUIRED
Towel or toweling mitts
Wide-tooth comb
Quartz or diffusion dryer
Hairdressing such as Vitapointe, or spray shine (optional)

CUTTING GUIDE

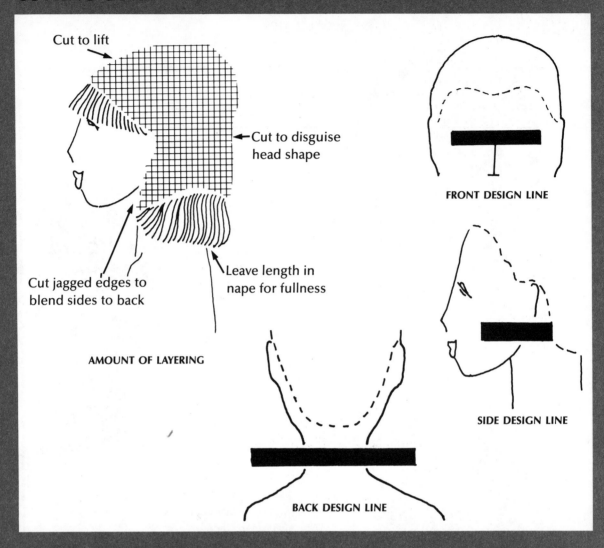

Cut to lift

Cut to disguise head shape

Cut jagged edges to blend sides to back

Leave length in nape for fullness

AMOUNT OF LAYERING

FRONT DESIGN LINE

SIDE DESIGN LINE

BACK DESIGN LINE

THIS STYLE HIDES

Head shape
Head size
Profile
Ears
Receding hairline
Low forehead
Narrow temples
Sparse hair at temples
Wide temples
Front hairline
Nape hairline
Neck shapes: wide,
   short, long, thin
Hair condition

THIS STYLE HIGHLIGHTS

Face shape
Chin
Jawline
Hairline in front of ears

BODY PROPORTIONS

Suitable for petite, small, medium, and tall proportions

THIS IS A *MINIMUM CARE* STYLE FOR WAVY-TO-CURLY HAIR.

THIS IS A *TEMPORARY* STYLE FOR STRAIGHT HAIR.

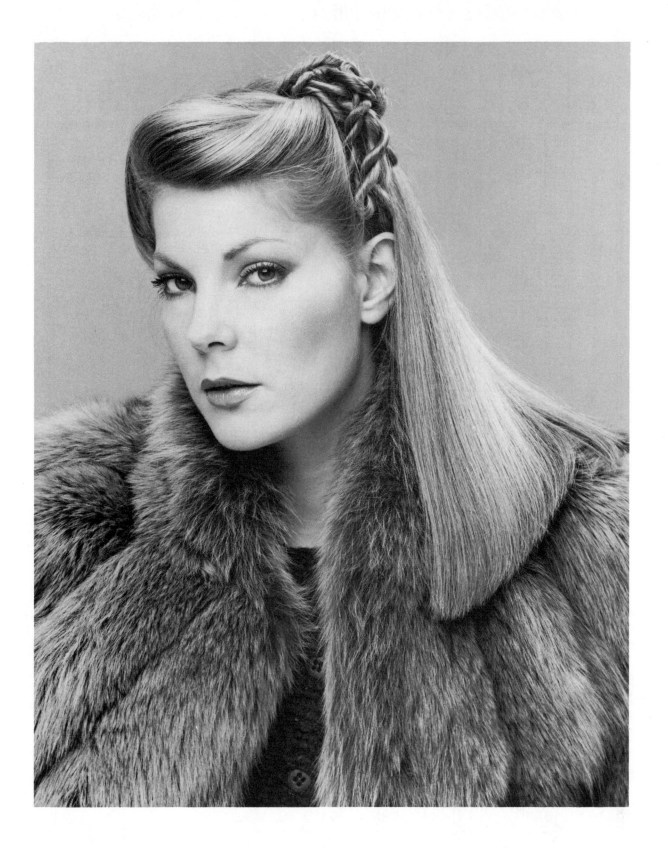

10 Dressed bob
for medium-to-long hair

Your Hair's Characteristics | Stylability

TEXTURE	FORMATION	QUANTITY	HAIR TYPE	CODE	TIMING*	SKILL RATING
FINE	STRAIGHT	THIN	1	C10 □	Drying time: 20 to 30 mins.; twisting time: 10 mins.	3 to 4
	STRAIGHT	MEDIUM	2	■		
	STRAIGHT	THICK	3	■		
	WAVY	THIN	4	C13 □		
	WAVY	MEDIUM	5	□		
	WAVY	THICK	6	□		
	CURLY	THIN	7	X		
	CURLY	MEDIUM	8	X		
	CURLY	THICK	9	X		
MEDIUM	STRAIGHT	THIN	10	C19 □	Drying time: 20 to 30 mins.; twisting time: 10 mins.	3 to 4
	STRAIGHT	MEDIUM	11	■		
	STRAIGHT	THICK	12	■		
	WAVY	THIN	13	C22 □		
	WAVY	MEDIUM	14	□		
	WAVY	THICK	15	□		
	CURLY	THIN	16	X		
	CURLY	MEDIUM	17	X		
	CURLY	THICK	18	X		
COARSE	STRAIGHT	THIN	19	C20 □	Drying time: 25 to 35 mins.; twisting time: 10 mins.	3 to 4
	STRAIGHT	MEDIUM	20	■		
	STRAIGHT	THICK	21	■		
	WAVY	THIN	22	C23 □		
	WAVY	MEDIUM	23	□		
	WAVY	THICK	24	□		
	CURLY	THIN	25	X		
	CURLY	MEDIUM	26	X		
	CURLY	THICK	27	X		

■ GOOD   □ POSSIBLE   X NOT RECOMMENDED   S STRAIGHTENING   C COLORING   WP WAVY PERM   CP CURLY PERM

*25% extra time for porous hair

Finishing and Styling Hints

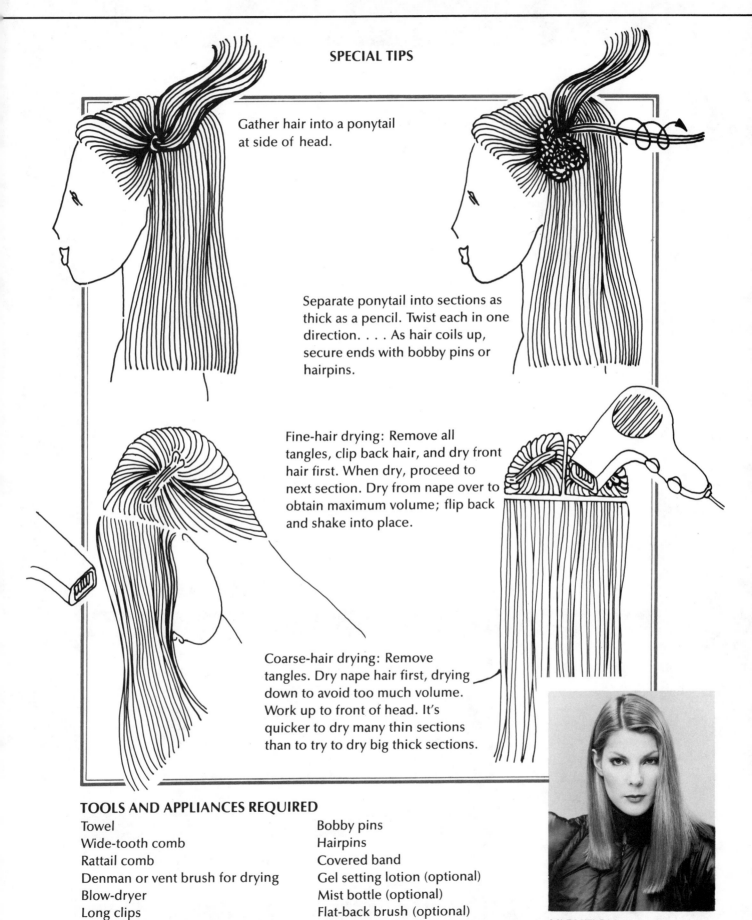

SPECIAL TIPS

Gather hair into a ponytail at side of head.

Separate ponytail into sections as thick as a pencil. Twist each in one direction. . . . As hair coils up, secure ends with bobby pins or hairpins.

Fine-hair drying: Remove all tangles, clip back hair, and dry front hair first. When dry, proceed to next section. Dry from nape over to obtain maximum volume; flip back and shake into place.

Coarse-hair drying: Remove tangles. Dry nape hair first, drying down to avoid too much volume. Work up to front of head. It's quicker to dry many thin sections than to try to dry big thick sections.

VARIATION

TOOLS AND APPLIANCES REQUIRED

Towel	Bobby pins
Wide-tooth comb	Hairpins
Rattail comb	Covered band
Denman or vent brush for drying	Gel setting lotion (optional)
Blow-dryer	Mist bottle (optional)
Long clips	Flat-back brush (optional)

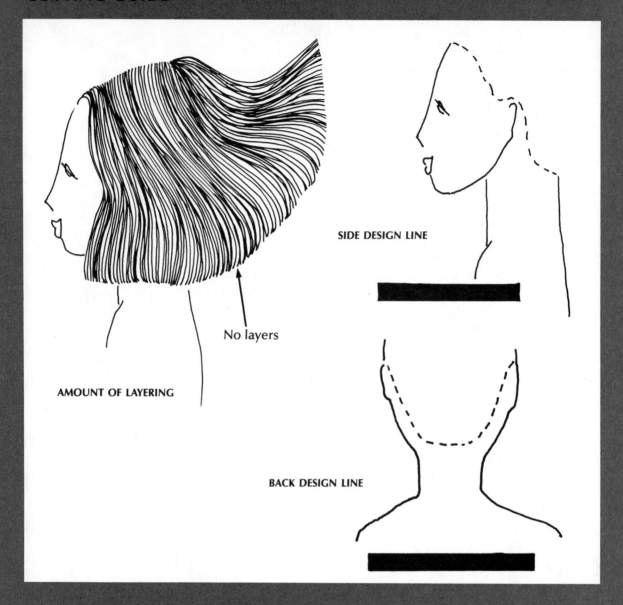

No layers

AMOUNT OF LAYERING

SIDE DESIGN LINE

BACK DESIGN LINE

THIS STYLE HIDES

Head shape
Nape hairline
Neck shapes: wide,
   short, long, thin

THIS STYLE HIGHLIGHTS

Profile
Nose
Ears
Face shape
Chin
Jawline

Receding hairline
Low forehead
Narrow temples
Sparse hair at temples
Wide temples
Front hairline
Hairline in front of ears
Hair condition

BODY PROPORTIONS
Suitable for all
proportions

THESE ARE *MINIMUM CARE* STYLES FOR STRAIGHT HAIR.

THESE ARE *TEMPORARY* STYLES FOR WAVY HAIR.

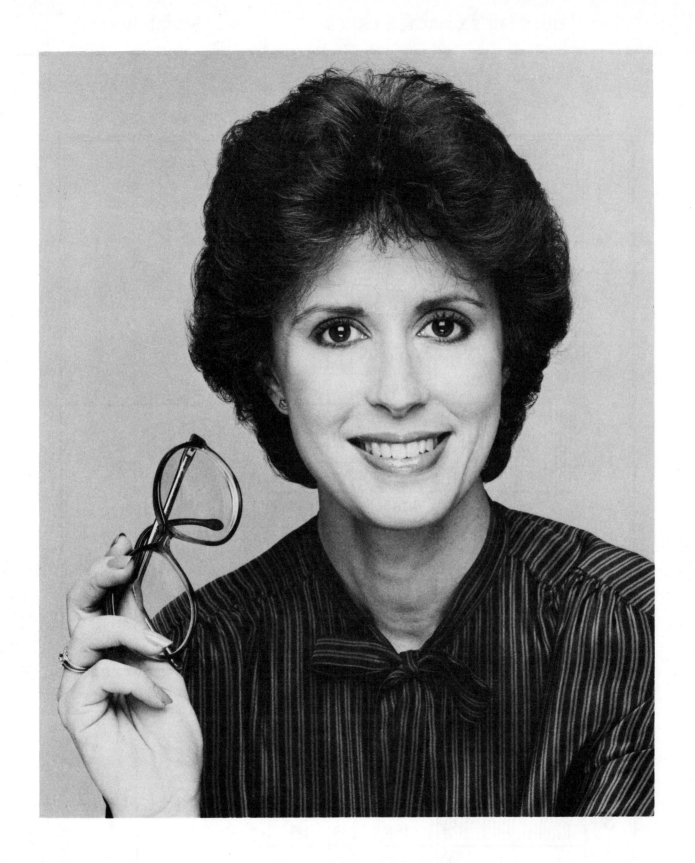

11 Classic cut for short hair

Your Hair's Characteristics | Stylability

TEXTURE	FORMATION	QUANTITY	HAIR TYPE	CODE	TIMING*	SKILL RATING
FINE	STRAIGHT	THIN	1	WP4 ■	25 to 30 mins.	3 to 4
FINE	STRAIGHT	MEDIUM	2	WP5 ■		
FINE	STRAIGHT	THICK	3	WP6 ■		
FINE	WAVY	THIN	4	C13 ■		
FINE	WAVY	MEDIUM	5	■		
FINE	WAVY	THICK	6	■		
FINE	CURLY	THIN	7	X		
FINE	CURLY	MEDIUM	8	X		
FINE	CURLY	THICK	9	S3 ■		
MEDIUM	STRAIGHT	THIN	10	WP13 ■	25 to 30 mins.	3 to 4
MEDIUM	STRAIGHT	MEDIUM	11	WP14 ■		
MEDIUM	STRAIGHT	THICK	12	WP15 ■		
MEDIUM	WAVY	THIN	13	C22 ■		
MEDIUM	WAVY	MEDIUM	14	■		
MEDIUM	WAVY	THICK	15	■		
MEDIUM	CURLY	THIN	16	S10 ■		
MEDIUM	CURLY	MEDIUM	17	S11 ■		
MEDIUM	CURLY	THICK	18	S12 ■		
COARSE	STRAIGHT	THIN	19	WP22 ■	25 to 30 mins.	3 to 4
COARSE	STRAIGHT	MEDIUM	20	WP23 ■		
COARSE	STRAIGHT	THICK	21	WP24 ■		
COARSE	WAVY	THIN	22	C23 ■		
COARSE	WAVY	MEDIUM	23	■		
COARSE	WAVY	THICK	24	■		
COARSE	CURLY	THIN	25	S19 ■		
COARSE	CURLY	MEDIUM	26	S20 ■		
COARSE	CURLY	THICK	27	S21 ■		

■ GOOD   □ POSSIBLE   X NOT RECOMMENDED   S STRAIGHTENING   C COLORING   WP WAVY PERM   CP CURLY PERM

*25% extra time for porous hair

Finishing and Styling Hints

SPECIAL TIPS

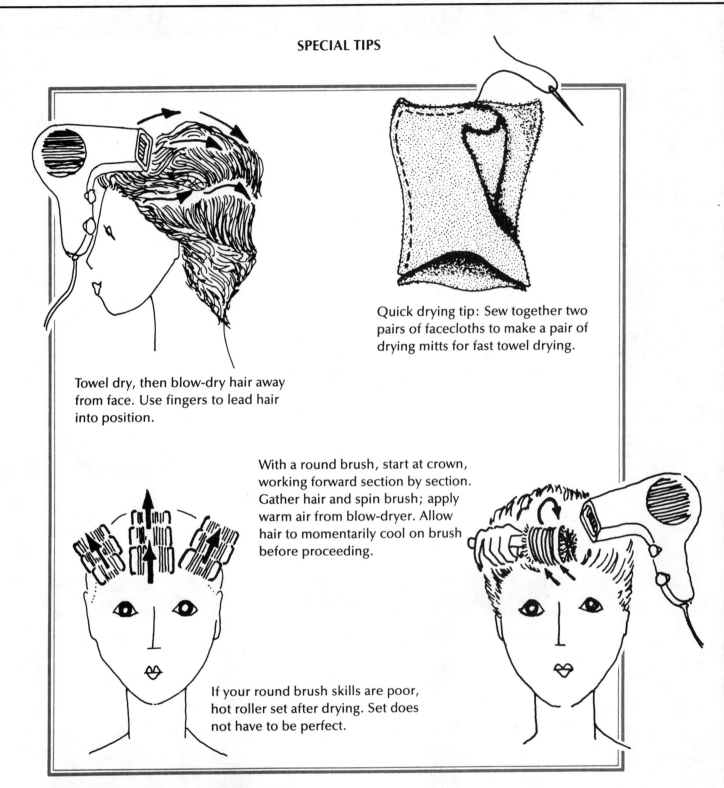

Towel dry, then blow-dry hair away from face. Use fingers to lead hair into position.

Quick drying tip: Sew together two pairs of facecloths to make a pair of drying mitts for fast towel drying.

With a round brush, start at crown, working forward section by section. Gather hair and spin brush; apply warm air from blow-dryer. Allow hair to momentarily cool on brush before proceeding.

If your round brush skills are poor, hot roller set after drying. Set does not have to be perfect.

TOOLS AND APPLIANCES REQUIRED
Towel or mitts
Wide-tooth comb
Rattail comb (if hot setting)
Large-diameter round brush and blow-dryer
or
Hot rollers and blow-dryer
Hair spray (optional)

CUTTING GUIDE

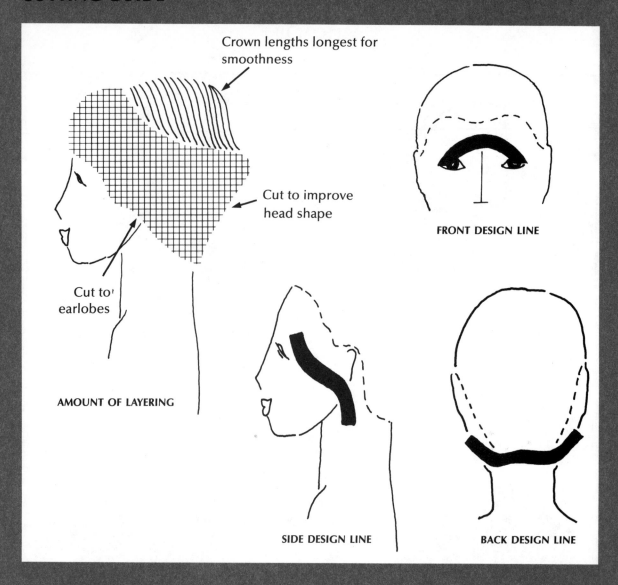

Crown lengths longest for smoothness

Cut to improve head shape

FRONT DESIGN LINE

Cut to earlobes

AMOUNT OF LAYERING

SIDE DESIGN LINE

BACK DESIGN LINE

THIS STYLE HIDES

Head shape
Head size
Profile
Ears
Wide face
Short face
Receding hairline
Low forehead
Narrow temples
Sparse hair at temples
Wide temples
Front hairline
Nape hairline
Short neck shape

THIS STYLE HIGHLIGHTS

Thin face
Long face
Chubby cheeks
Chin
Jawline
Hairline in front of ears
Wide neck
Hair condition

BODY PROPORTIONS

Suitable for small, medium, and tall proportions

THIS IS A *MINIMUM CARE* STYLE FOR STRAIGHT AND WAVY HAIR.

THIS IS A *TEMPORARY* STYLE FOR CURLY HAIR.

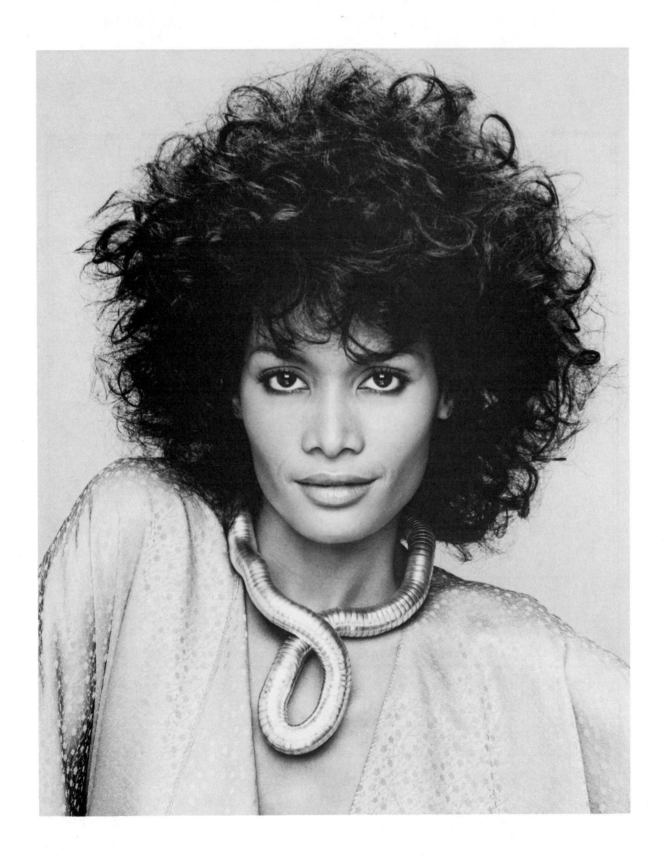

12 Liberty curl

Your Hair's Characteristics | Stylability

TEXTURE	FORMATION	QUANTITY	HAIR TYPE	CODE	TIMING	SKILL RATING
FINE	STRAIGHT	THIN	1	CP7 ■	**Note:** This style does not require freshly shampooed hair. Time estimates are for dry-hair styling. 15 to 25 mins.	3 to 4
	STRAIGHT	MEDIUM	2	CP8 ■		
	STRAIGHT	THICK	3	CP9 ■		
	WAVY	THIN	4	C13 ☐		
	WAVY	MEDIUM	5	☐		
	WAVY	THICK	6	☐		
	CURLY	THIN	7	C16 ■		
	CURLY	MEDIUM	8	■		
	CURLY	THICK	9	■		
MEDIUM	STRAIGHT	THIN	10	CP16 ■	20 to 30 mins.	3 to 4
	STRAIGHT	MEDIUM	11	CP17 ■		
	STRAIGHT	THICK	12	CP18 ■		
	WAVY	THIN	13	C22 ☐		
	WAVY	MEDIUM	14	☐		
	WAVY	THICK	15	☐		
	CURLY	THIN	16	C25 ■		
	CURLY	MEDIUM	17	■		
	CURLY	THICK	18	■		
COARSE	STRAIGHT	THIN	19	CP25 ■	20 to 30 mins.	3 to 4
	STRAIGHT	MEDIUM	20	CP26 ■		
	STRAIGHT	THICK	21	CP27 ■		
	WAVY	THIN	22	C23 ☐		
	WAVY	MEDIUM	23	☐		
	WAVY	THICK	24	☐		
	CURLY	THIN	25	C26 ■		
	CURLY	MEDIUM	26	■		
	CURLY	THICK	27	■		

■ GOOD   ☐ POSSIBLE   X NOT RECOMMENDED   S STRAIGHTENING   C COLORING   WP WAVY PERM   CP CURLY PERM

Finishing and Styling Hints

SPECIAL TIPS

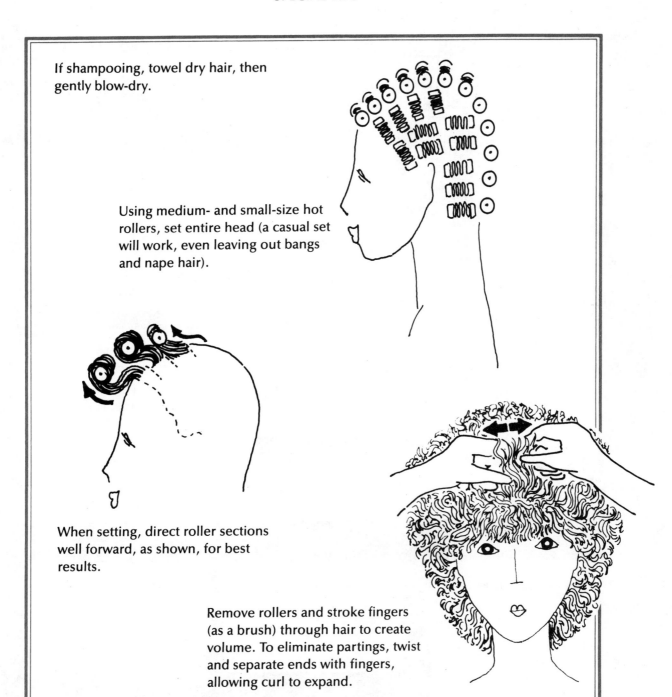

If shampooing, towel dry hair, then gently blow-dry.

Using medium- and small-size hot rollers, set entire head (a casual set will work, even leaving out bangs and nape hair).

When setting, direct roller sections well forward, as shown, for best results.

Remove rollers and stroke fingers (as a brush) through hair to create volume. To eliminate partings, twist and separate ends with fingers, allowing curl to expand.

TOOLS AND APPLIANCES REQUIRED
Towel
Wide-tooth comb
Rattail comb
Blow-dryer
Hot rollers
Spray shine or hairdressing, such as Vitapointe (optional)

CUTTING GUIDE

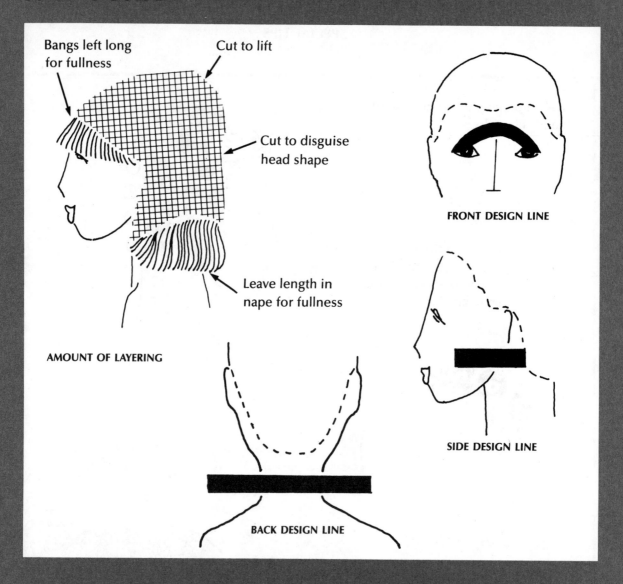

Bangs left long for fullness

Cut to lift

Cut to disguise head shape

Leave length in nape for fullness

AMOUNT OF LAYERING

FRONT DESIGN LINE

SIDE DESIGN LINE

BACK DESIGN LINE

THIS STYLE HIDES

Head shape
Head size
Profile
Low forehead
Front hairline
Nape hairline
Short neck
Ears
Hairline in front of ears

THIS STYLE HIGHLIGHTS

Face shape
Chin
Jawline

BODY PROPORTIONS

Suitable for medium, tall, and large proportions

THIS IS A *MINIMUM CARE* STYLE FOR CURLY-TO-WAVY HAIR.

THIS IS A *TEMPORARY* STYLE FOR STRAIGHT HAIR.

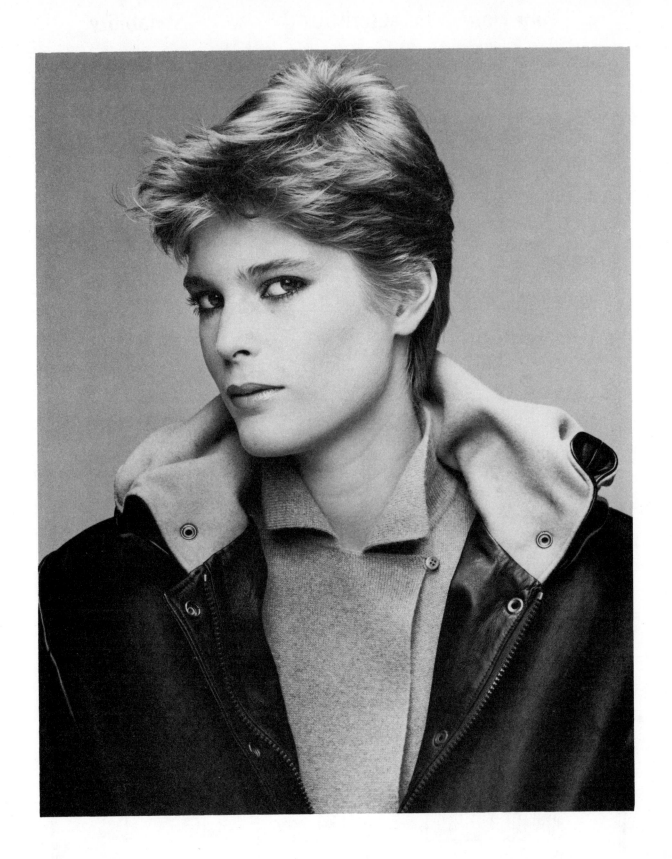

13 Splinters for effect

Your Hair's Characteristics | Stylability

TEXTURE	FORMATION	QUANTITY	HAIR TYPE	CODE	TIMING*	SKILL RATING
FINE	STRAIGHT	THIN	1	C10 ■	10 to 15 mins.	1 to 2
		MEDIUM	2	C11 ■		
		THICK	3	■		
	WAVY	THIN	4	C13 □		
		MEDIUM	5	□		
		THICK	6	□		
	CURLY	THIN	7	X		
		MEDIUM	8	X		
		THICK	9	S3 ■		
MEDIUM	STRAIGHT	THIN	10	C19 ■	10 to 15 mins.	1 to 2
		MEDIUM	11	■		
		THICK	12	■		
	WAVY	THIN	13	C22 □		
		MEDIUM	14	□		
		THICK	15	□		
	CURLY	THIN	16	S10 ■		
		MEDIUM	17	S11 ■		
		THICK	18	S12 ■		
COARSE	STRAIGHT	THIN	19	C20 ■	10 to 15 mins.	1 to 2
		MEDIUM	20	■		
		THICK	21	■		
	WAVY	THIN	22	C23 □		
		MEDIUM	23	□		
		THICK	24	□		
	CURLY	THIN	25	S19 ■		
		MEDIUM	26	S20 ■		
		THICK	27	S21 ■		

■ GOOD   □ POSSIBLE   X NOT RECOMMENDED   S STRAIGHTENING   C COLORING   WP WAVY PERM   CP CURLY PERM

140

*25% extra time for porous hair

Finishing and Styling Hints

SPECIAL TIPS

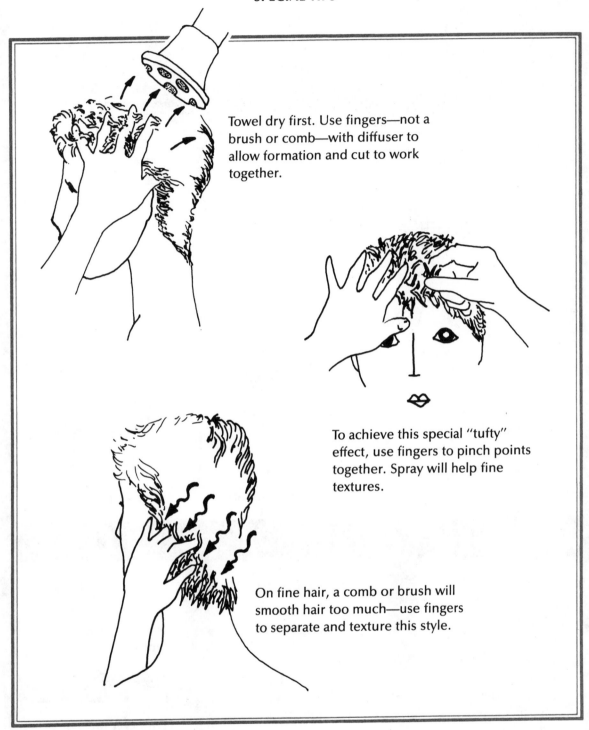

Towel dry first. Use fingers—not a brush or comb—with diffuser to allow formation and cut to work together.

To achieve this special "tufty" effect, use fingers to pinch points together. Spray will help fine textures.

On fine hair, a comb or brush will smooth hair too much—use fingers to separate and texture this style.

TOOLS AND APPLIANCES REQUIRED
Towel
Quartz or diffusion dryer
Hair spray (optional)

CUTTING GUIDE

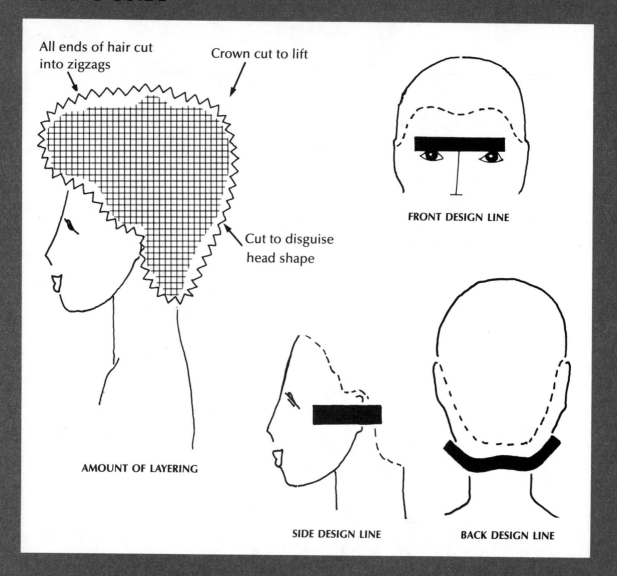

All ends of hair cut into zigzags

Crown cut to lift

Cut to disguise head shape

AMOUNT OF LAYERING

FRONT DESIGN LINE

SIDE DESIGN LINE

BACK DESIGN LINE

THIS STYLE HIDES

Head shape
Head size
Profile
Receding hairline
Low forehead
Narrow temples
Sparse hair at temples
Wide temples
Front hairline
Nape hairline

THIS STYLE HIGHLIGHTS

Ears
Face shape
Chin
Jawline
Hairline in front of ears
Neck shapes: wide,
    short, long, thin
Hair condition

BODY PROPORTIONS

Suitable for petite, small, and medium proportions

THIS IS A *MINIMUM CARE* STYLE FOR STRAIGHT AND WAVY HAIR.

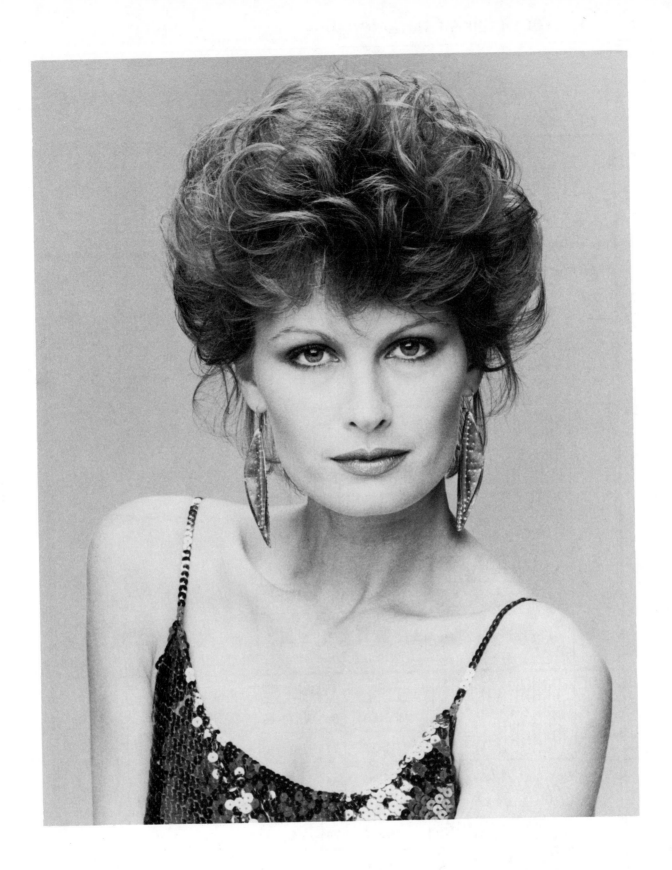

14   Fine finesse

Your Hair's Characteristics | Stylability

TEXTURE	FORMATION	QUANTITY	HAIR TYPE	CODE	TIMING*	SKILL RATING
FINE	STRAIGHT	THIN	1	WP4 ◼	25 to 30 mins.	3 to 4
		MEDIUM	2	WP5 ◼		
		THICK	3	WP6 ◼		
	WAVY	THIN	4	C13 ◼		
		MEDIUM	5	◼		
		THICK	6	◼		
	CURLY	THIN	7	C16 ☐		
		MEDIUM	8	☐		
		THICK	9	☐		
MEDIUM	STRAIGHT	THIN	10	WP13 ◼	25 to 30 mins.	3 to 4
		MEDIUM	11	WP14 ◼		
		THICK	12	WP15 ◼		
	WAVY	THIN	13	C22 ◼		
		MEDIUM	14	◼		
		THICK	15	◼		
	CURLY	THIN	16	C25 ☐		
		MEDIUM	17	☐		
		THICK	18	☐		
COARSE	STRAIGHT	THIN	19	WP22 ◼	30 to 35 mins.	3 to 4
		MEDIUM	20	WP23 ◼		
		THICK	21	WP24 ◼		
	WAVY	THIN	22	◼		
		MEDIUM	23	◼		
		THICK	24	◼		
	CURLY	THIN	25	C26 ☐		
		MEDIUM	26	☐		
		THICK	27	☐		

144

◼ GOOD ☐ POSSIBLE X NOT RECOMMENDED

S STRAIGHTENING C COLORING WP WAVY PERM CP CURLY PERM

*25% extra time for porous hair

Finishing and Styling Hints

SPECIAL TIPS

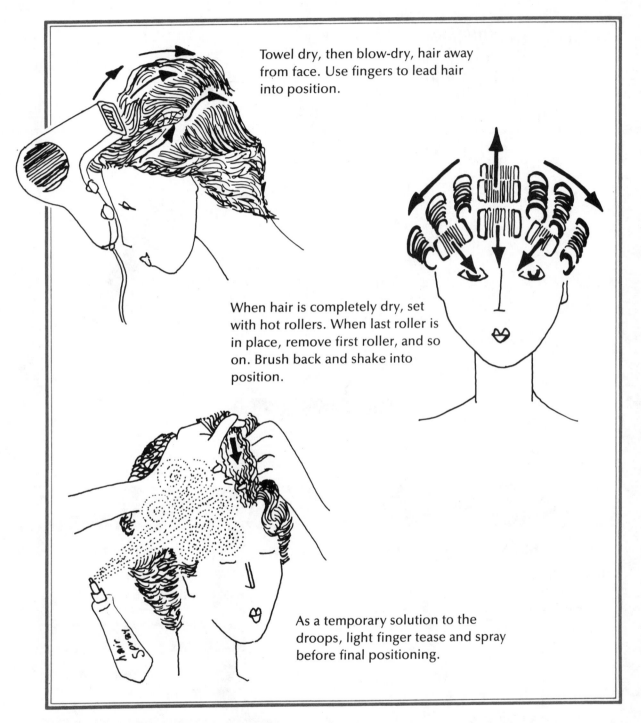

Towel dry, then blow-dry, hair away from face. Use fingers to lead hair into position.

When hair is completely dry, set with hot rollers. When last roller is in place, remove first roller, and so on. Brush back and shake into position.

As a temporary solution to the droops, light finger tease and spray before final positioning.

TOOLS AND APPLIANCES REQUIRED
Towel
Wide-tooth comb
Rattail comb
Denman or vent brush
Blow-dryer
Hot rollers
Hair spray (optional)

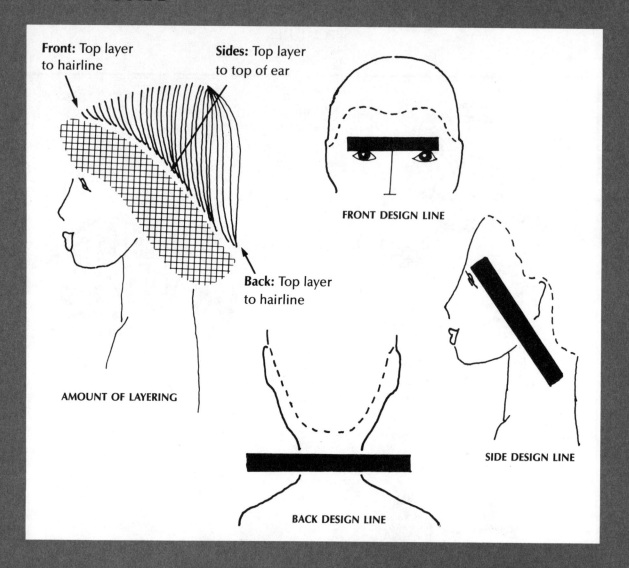

Front: Top layer to hairline

Sides: Top layer to top of ear

Back: Top layer to hairline

AMOUNT OF LAYERING

FRONT DESIGN LINE

SIDE DESIGN LINE

BACK DESIGN LINE

THIS STYLE HIDES

Head shape
Hair condition
Low nape hairline
Low forehead

THIS STYLE HIGHLIGHTS

Short face
Chin
Jawline
Hairline in front of ears

BODY PROPORTIONS

Suitable for medium and tall proportions

THIS IS A *TEMPORARY* STYLE.

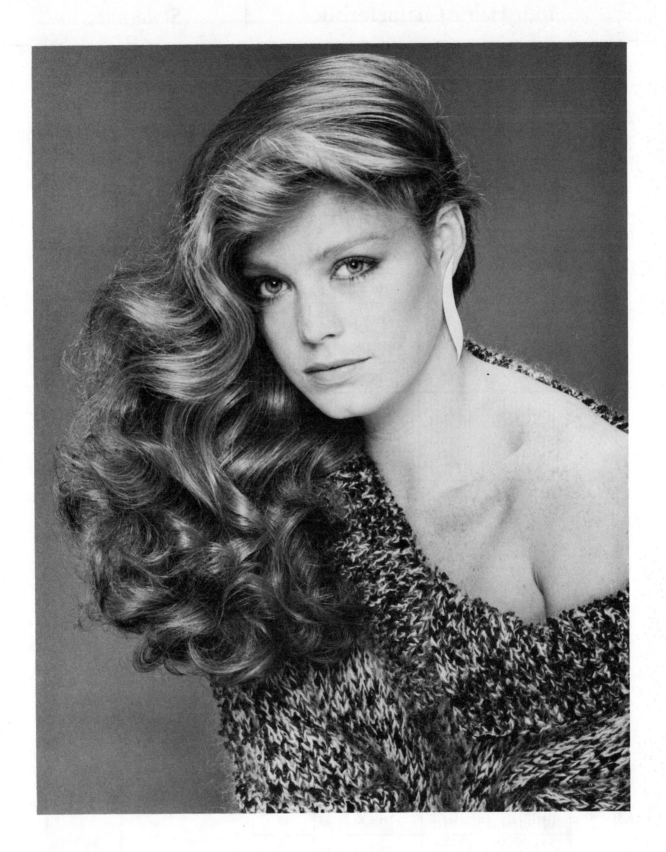

15 Luxurious length
with bounce and body

Your Hair's Characteristics

Stylability

TEXTURE	FORMATION	QUANTITY	HAIR TYPE	CODE	TIMING*	SKILL RATING
FINE	STRAIGHT	THIN	1	WP4 ■	**Note:** This style does not require freshly shampooed hair. 30 to 40 mins.; if setting only, 10 to 20 mins.	3 to 4
	STRAIGHT	MEDIUM	2	WP5 ■		
	STRAIGHT	THICK	3	WP6 ■		
	WAVY	THIN	4	C13 ■		
	WAVY	MEDIUM	5	■		
	WAVY	THICK	6	■		
	CURLY	THIN	7	□		
	CURLY	MEDIUM	8	□		
	CURLY	THICK	9	□		
MEDIUM	STRAIGHT	THIN	10	WP13 ■	35 to 45 mins.; if setting only, 10 to 20 mins.	3 to 4
	STRAIGHT	MEDIUM	11	WP14 ■		
	STRAIGHT	THICK	12	WP15 ■		
	WAVY	THIN	13	C22 ■		
	WAVY	MEDIUM	14	■		
	WAVY	THICK	15	■		
	CURLY	THIN	16	□		
	CURLY	MEDIUM	17	□		
	CURLY	THICK	18	□		
COARSE	STRAIGHT	THIN	19	WP22 ■	40 to 50 mins.; if setting only, 10 to 20 mins.	3 to 4
	STRAIGHT	MEDIUM	20	WP23 ■		
	STRAIGHT	THICK	21	WP24 ■		
	WAVY	THIN	22	C23 ■		
	WAVY	MEDIUM	23	■		
	WAVY	THICK	24	■		
	CURLY	THIN	25	□		
	CURLY	MEDIUM	26	□		
	CURLY	THICK	27	□		

148

■ GOOD   □ POSSIBLE   X NOT RECOMMENDED   **S** STRAIGHTENING   **C** COLORING   **WP** WAVY PERM   **CP** CURLY PERM

*25% extra time for porous hair

Finishing and Styling Hints

SPECIAL TIPS

Using a covered band and two bobby pins, secure a bobby pin at base of tail, move band around, and secure with second bobby.

Note: Even a covered band will often break fine hair. By releasing bobby pins, band will fall harmlessly from hair.

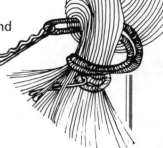

Towel dry, then gently blow-dry, hair. Gather into a ponytail using a covered band and bobby pins.

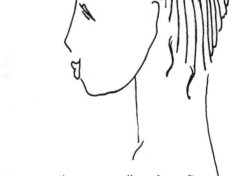

Set ponytail—many rollers for a firm result, few rollers for a soft result.

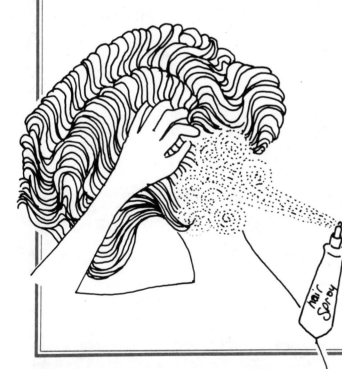

For extra volume, lean forward; spray underneath sections to give lift to your style.

TOOLS AND APPLIANCES REQUIRED

Towel	Hot rollers
Wide-tooth comb	Long clips
Rattail comb	Covered band with bobby pins
Denman brush	Antistatic material (for fine textures)
Blow-dryer	Hair spray (optional)

CUTTING GUIDE

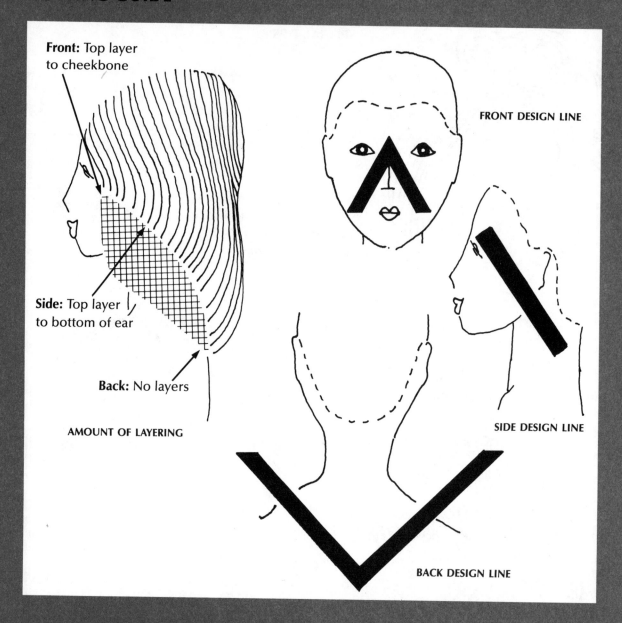

Front: Top layer to cheekbone

Side: Top layer to bottom of ear

Back: No layers

AMOUNT OF LAYERING

FRONT DESIGN LINE

SIDE DESIGN LINE

BACK DESIGN LINE

THIS STYLE HIDES

Head size
Profile
Wide face
Chin and jawline
Neck shapes: wide,
  short, long, or thin

THIS STYLE HIGHLIGHTS

Hair condition
Long face

BODY PROPORTIONS

Suitable for medium,
tall, and large
proportions

THIS IS A *MINIMUM CARE* STYLE FOR WAVY HAIR.

THIS IS A *TEMPORARY* STYLE FOR STRAIGHT HAIR.

150

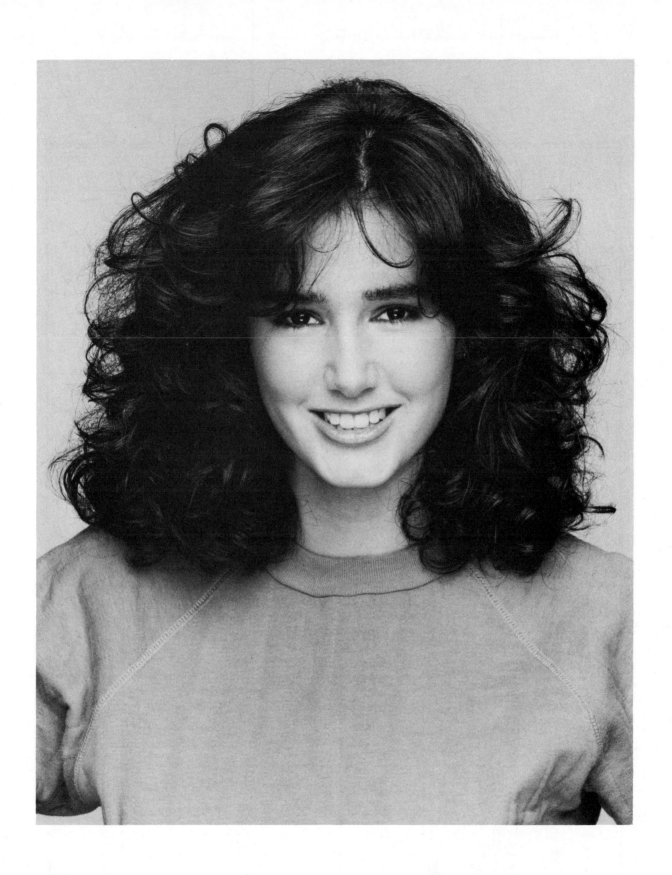

16 The sweet, savage look

Your Hair's Characteristics | Stylability

TEXTURE	FORMATION	QUANTITY	HAIR TYPE	CODE	TIMING*	SKILL RATING
FINE	STRAIGHT	THIN	1	WP4 ■	30 to 40 mins.	2 to 3
		MEDIUM	2	WP5 ■		
		THICK	3	WP6 ■		
	WAVY	THIN	4	C13 ■		
		MEDIUM	5	■		
		THICK	6	■		
	CURLY	THIN	7	C16 ■		
		MEDIUM	8	☐		
		THICK	9	☐		
MEDIUM	STRAIGHT	THIN	10	WP13 ■	30 to 40 mins.	2 to 3
		MEDIUM	11	WP14 ■		
		THICK	12	WP15 ■		
	WAVY	THIN	13	C22 ■		
		MEDIUM	14	■		
		THICK	15	■		
	CURLY	THIN	16	C25 ☐		
		MEDIUM	17	☐		
		THICK	18	☐		
COARSE	STRAIGHT	THIN	19	WP22 ■	30 to 40 mins.	2 to 3
		MEDIUM	20	WP23 ■		
		THICK	21	WP24 ■		
	WAVY	THIN	22	C23 ■		
		MEDIUM	23	■		
		THICK	24	■		
	CURLY	THIN	25	C26 ☐		
		MEDIUM	26	☐		
		THICK	27	☐		

■ GOOD   ☐ POSSIBLE   X NOT RECOMMENDED   S STRAIGHTENING   C COLORING   WP WAVY PERM   CP CURLY PERM

152

*25% extra time for porous hair

Finishing and Styling Hints

SPECIAL TIPS

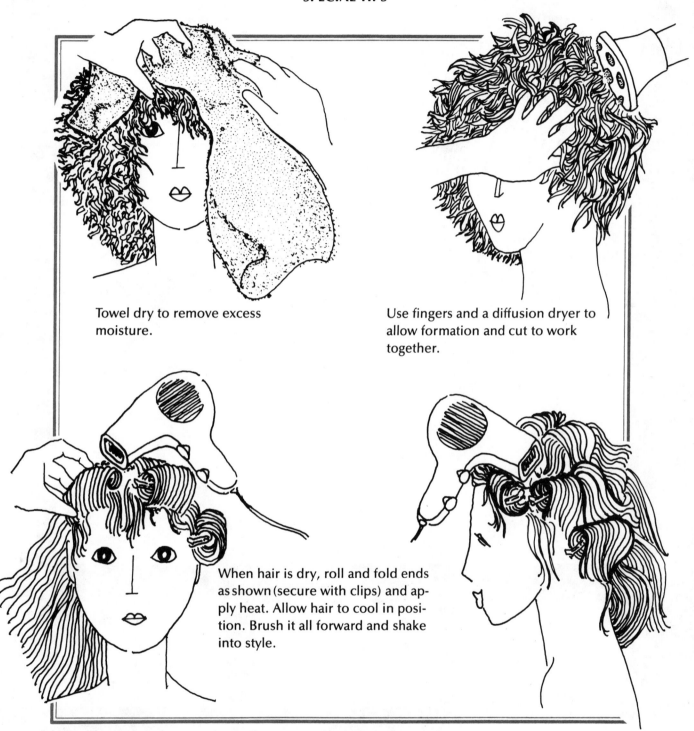

Towel dry to remove excess moisture.

Use fingers and a diffusion dryer to allow formation and cut to work together.

When hair is dry, roll and fold ends as shown (secure with clips) and apply heat. Allow hair to cool in position. Brush it all forward and shake into style.

TOOLS AND APPLIANCES REQUIRED

Towel	Short clips
Wide-tooth comb	Mist bottle
Quartz or diffusion dryer	Antistatic material (for fine textures)
Blow-dryer	Hair spray (optional)

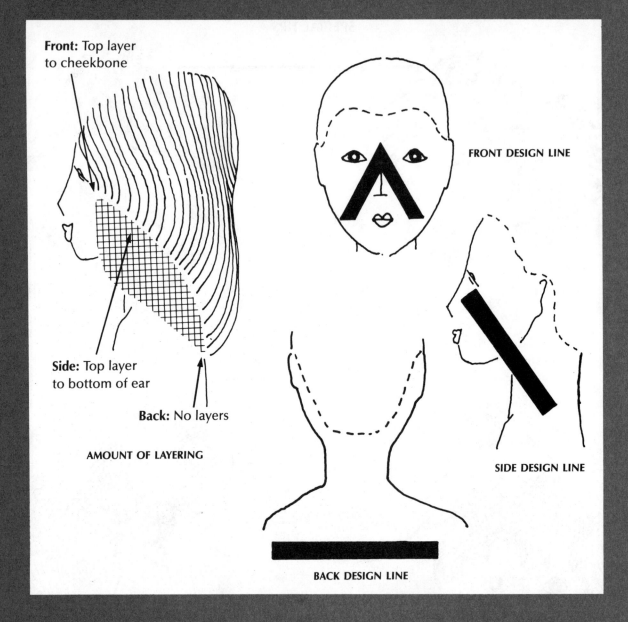

Front: Top layer to cheekbone

Side: Top layer to bottom of ear

Back: No layers

AMOUNT OF LAYERING

FRONT DESIGN LINE

SIDE DESIGN LINE

BACK DESIGN LINE

THIS STYLE HIDES

Head shape
Head size
Profile
Ears
Face shape
Chin
Jawline
All hairlines
Neck shapes: wide,
    short, long, thin

THIS STYLE HIGHLIGHTS

Hair condition

BODY PROPORTIONS

Suitable for small,
medium, large,
and tall proportions

THIS IS A *MINIMUM CARE* STYLE FOR WAVY-TO-CURLY HAIR.

THIS IS A *TEMPORARY* STYLE FOR STRAIGHT HAIR.

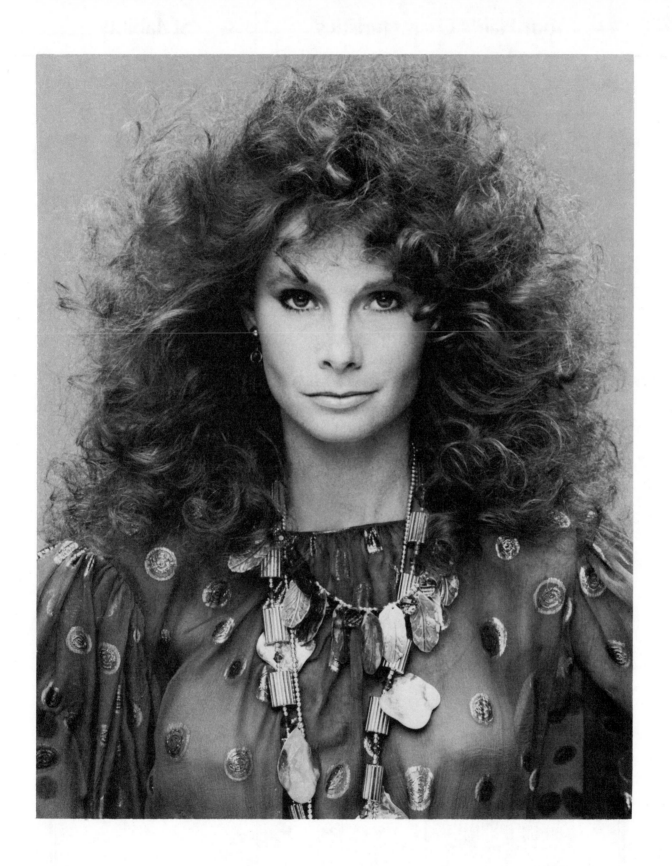

17 Voluptuous curls

Your Hair's Characteristics | Stylability

TEXTURE	FORMATION	QUANTITY	HAIR TYPE	CODE	TIMING*	SKILL RATING
FINE	STRAIGHT	THIN	1	WP4 ■	35 to 40 mins.	3 to 4
		MEDIUM	2	WP5 ■		
		THICK	3	WP6 ■		
	WAVY	THIN	4	C13 ■		
		MEDIUM	5	C14 ■		
		THICK	6	■		
	CURLY	THIN	7	C16 □		
		MEDIUM	8	□		
		THICK	9	□		
MEDIUM	STRAIGHT	THIN	10	WP13 ■	35 to 40 mins.	3 to 4
		MEDIUM	11	WP14 ■		
		THICK	12	WP15 ■		
	WAVY	THIN	13	C22 ■		
		MEDIUM	14	■		
		THICK	15	■		
	CURLY	THIN	16	C25 □		
		MEDIUM	17	□		
		THICK	18	□		
COARSE	STRAIGHT	THIN	19	WP22 ■	35 to 50 mins.	3 to 4
		MEDIUM	20	WP23 ■		
		THICK	21	WP24 ■		
	WAVY	THIN	22	C23 ■		
		MEDIUM	23	■		
		THICK	24	■		
	CURLY	THIN	25	□		
		MEDIUM	26	□		
		THICK	27	□		

■ GOOD □ POSSIBLE X NOT RECOMMENDED   S STRAIGHTENING C COLORING WP WAVY PERM CP CURLY PERM

*25% extra time for porous hair

Finishing and Styling Hints

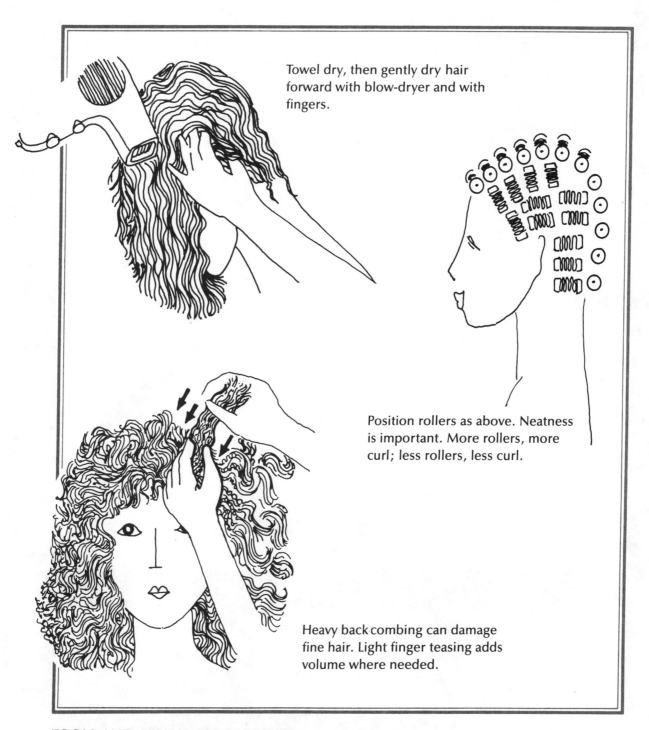

Towel dry, then gently dry hair forward with blow-dryer and with fingers.

Position rollers as above. Neatness is important. More rollers, more curl; less rollers, less curl.

Heavy back combing can damage fine hair. Light finger teasing adds volume where needed.

TOOLS AND APPLIANCES REQUIRED

Towel
Wide-tooth comb
Rattail comb
Vent brush

Blow-dryer
Hot rollers
Hair spray (optional)
Spray shine (optional)

CUTTING GUIDE

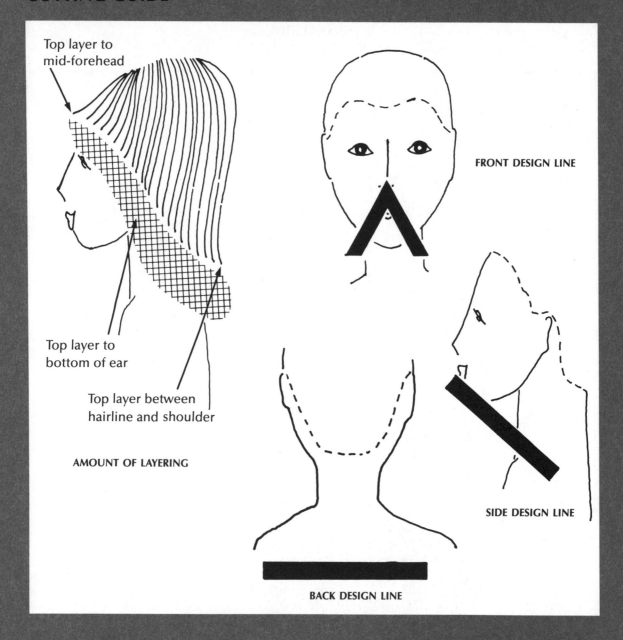

Top layer to mid-forehead

Top layer to bottom of ear

Top layer between hairline and shoulder

AMOUNT OF LAYERING

FRONT DESIGN LINE

SIDE DESIGN LINE

BACK DESIGN LINE

THIS STYLE HIDES

Head shape
Head size
Profile
Ears
Face shape
Chubby cheeks
Chin
Jawline
All hairlines
Neck shapes: wide,
    short, long, thin

THIS STYLE HIGHLIGHTS

Hair condition

BODY PROPORTIONS

Suitable for medium, tall, and large proportions

THIS IS A *MINIMUM CARE* STYLE FOR WAVY-TO-CURLY HAIR.

THIS IS A *TEMPORARY* STYLE FOR STRAIGHT HAIR.

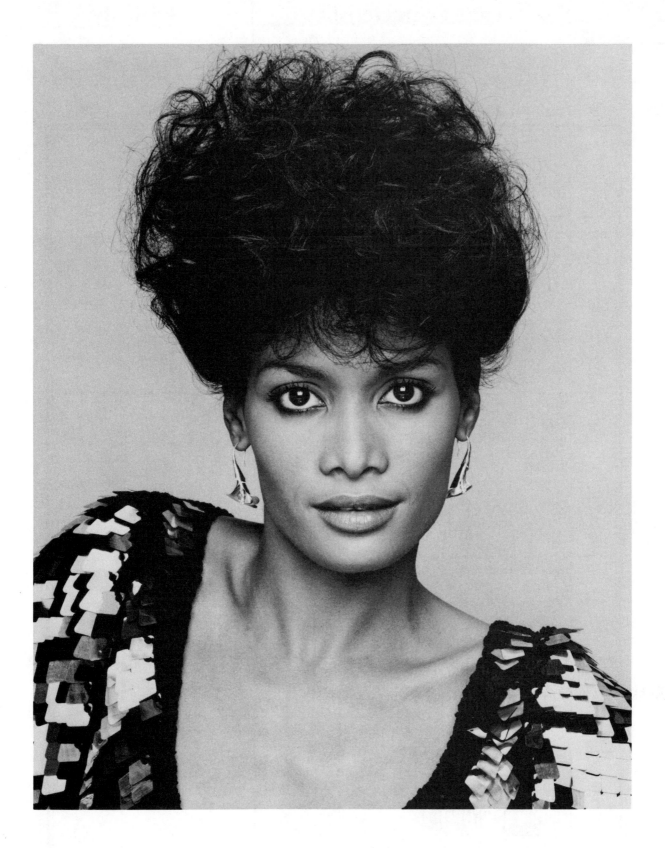

18 Positioning curls for a dramatic evening look

Your Hair's Characteristics | Stylability

TEXTURE	FORMATION	QUANTITY	HAIR TYPE	CODE	TIMING	SKILL RATING
FINE	STRAIGHT	THIN	1	WP4 ■	**Note:** This style does not require freshly shampooed hair. Time estimates are for dry-hair styling.	3
	STRAIGHT	MEDIUM	2	WP5 ■		
	STRAIGHT	THICK	3	WP6 ■		
	WAVY	THIN	4	C13 ■		
	WAVY	MEDIUM	5	■	10 to 20 mins.	
	WAVY	THICK	6	■		
	CURLY	THIN	7	C16 ■		
	CURLY	MEDIUM	8	■		
	CURLY	THICK	9	■		
MEDIUM	STRAIGHT	THIN	10	WP13 ■		3
	STRAIGHT	MEDIUM	11	WP14 ■		
	STRAIGHT	THICK	12	WP15 ■		
	WAVY	THIN	13	C22 ■	10 to 20 mins.	
	WAVY	MEDIUM	14	■		
	WAVY	THICK	15	■		
	CURLY	THIN	16	C25 ■		
	CURLY	MEDIUM	17	■		
	CURLY	THICK	18	■		
COARSE	STRAIGHT	THIN	19	WP22 ■		3
	STRAIGHT	MEDIUM	20	WP23 ■		
	STRAIGHT	THICK	21	WP24 ■		
	WAVY	THIN	22	C23 ■	10 to 20 mins.	
	WAVY	MEDIUM	23	■		
	WAVY	THICK	24	■		
	CURLY	THIN	25	C26 ■		
	CURLY	MEDIUM	26	■		
	CURLY	THICK	27	■		

■ GOOD ☐ POSSIBLE X NOT RECOMMENDED S STRAIGHTENING C COLORING WP WAVY PERM CP CURLY PERM

160

Finishing and Styling Hints

SPECIAL TIPS

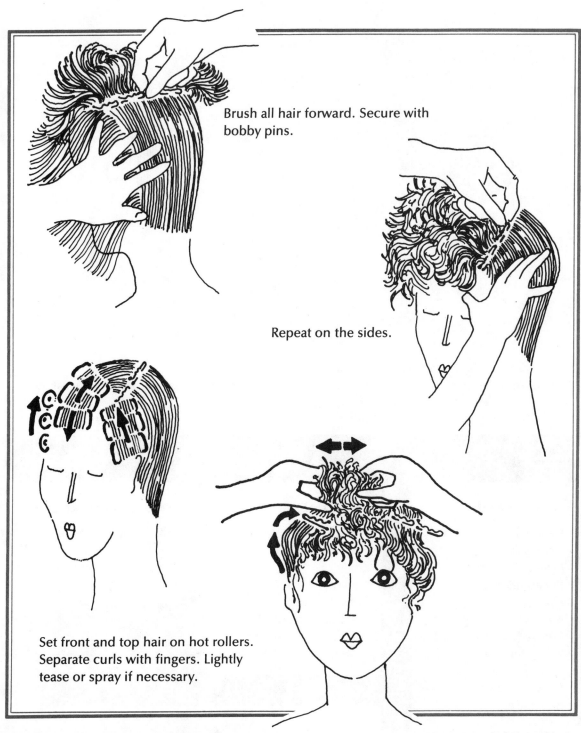

Brush all hair forward. Secure with bobby pins.

Repeat on the sides.

Set front and top hair on hot rollers. Separate curls with fingers. Lightly tease or spray if necessary.

TOOLS AND APPLIANCES REQUIRED

Wide-tooth comb	Hairpins
Rattail comb	Flat-back brush
Hot rollers	Spray shine (optional)
Bobby pins	Hair spray (optional)

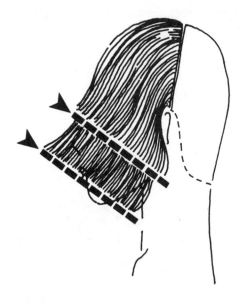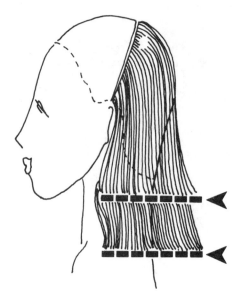

MINIMUM LENGTHS REQUIRED

Front: Top layers at least over brow. Bottom lengths at least below nose.

Back: Top layer at least over hairline. Bottom length at least to shoulder.

THIS STYLE HIDES

Head shape
Head size
Profile
Receding hairline
Low forehead
Narrow temples
Sparse hair at temples
Wide temples
Front hairline
Hair condition
Bad haircut

THIS STYLE HIGHLIGHTS

Ears
Face shape
Chin
Jawline
Nape hairline
Hairline in front of ears
Neck shapes: wide,
    short, long, thin

BODY PROPORTIONS

Suitable for petite, small, medium, and tall proportions

THIS IS A *MINIMUM CARE* STYLE FOR CURLY AND WAVY HAIR.

THIS IS A *TEMPORARY* STYLE FOR STRAIGHT HAIR.

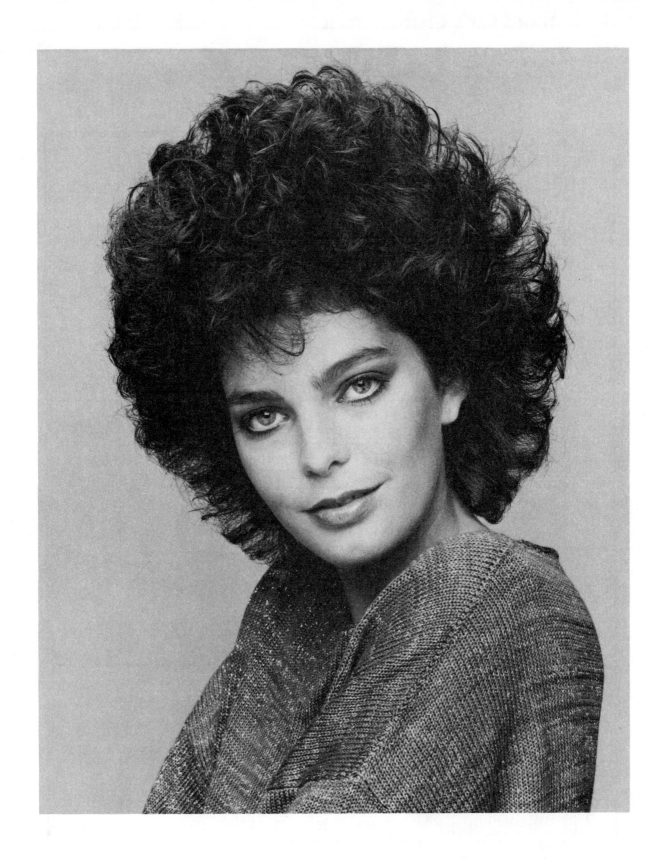

19 Contemporary curl

Your Hair's Characteristics | Stylability

TEXTURE	FORMATION	QUANTITY	HAIR TYPE	CODE	TIMING*	SKILL RATING
FINE	STRAIGHT	THIN	1	CP7 ■		
FINE	STRAIGHT	MEDIUM	2	CP8 ■		
FINE	STRAIGHT	THICK	3	CP9 ■		
FINE	WAVY	THIN	4	CP7 □		
FINE	WAVY	MEDIUM	5	□	20 to 30 mins.	2 to 3
FINE	WAVY	THICK	6	□		
FINE	CURLY	THIN	7	C16 ■		
FINE	CURLY	MEDIUM	8	■		
FINE	CURLY	THICK	9	■		
MEDIUM	STRAIGHT	THIN	10	CP16 ■		
MEDIUM	STRAIGHT	MEDIUM	11	CP17 ■		
MEDIUM	STRAIGHT	THICK	12	CP18 ■		
MEDIUM	WAVY	THIN	13	C22 □		
MEDIUM	WAVY	MEDIUM	14	□	20 to 30 mins.	2 to 3
MEDIUM	WAVY	THICK	15	□		
MEDIUM	CURLY	THIN	16	■		
MEDIUM	CURLY	MEDIUM	17	■		
MEDIUM	CURLY	THICK	18	■		
COARSE	STRAIGHT	THIN	19	CP25 ■		
COARSE	STRAIGHT	MEDIUM	20	CP26 ■		
COARSE	STRAIGHT	THICK	21	CP27 ■		
COARSE	WAVY	THIN	22	C23 □		
COARSE	WAVY	MEDIUM	23	□	20 to 30 mins.	2 to 3
COARSE	WAVY	THICK	24	□		
COARSE	CURLY	THIN	25	■		
COARSE	CURLY	MEDIUM	26	■		
COARSE	CURLY	THICK	27	■		

■ GOOD   □ POSSIBLE   X NOT RECOMMENDED   S STRAIGHTENING   C COLORING   WP WAVY PERM   CP CURLY PERM

164

*25% extra time for porous hair

Finishing and Styling Hints

SPECIAL TIPS

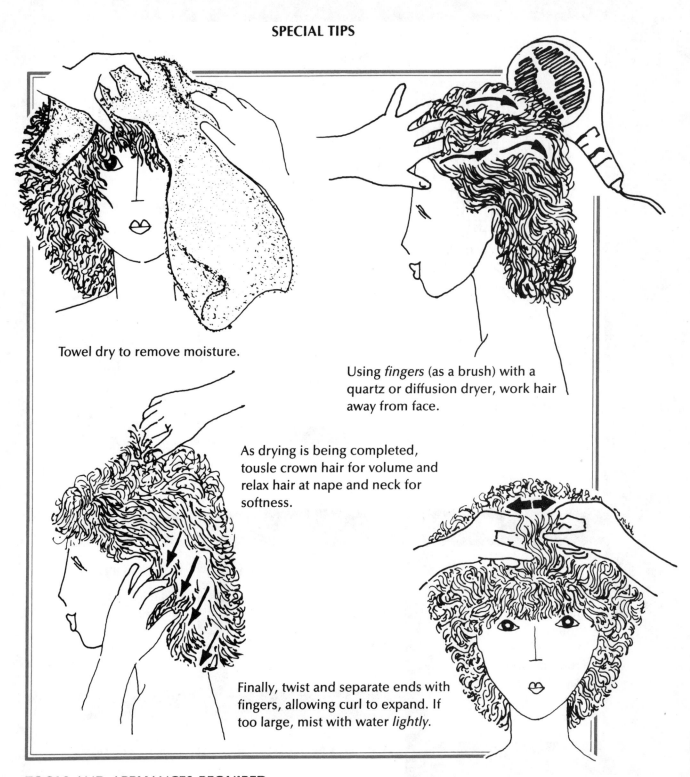

Towel dry to remove moisture.

Using *fingers* (as a brush) with a quartz or diffusion dryer, work hair away from face.

As drying is being completed, tousle crown hair for volume and relax hair at nape and neck for softness.

Finally, twist and separate ends with fingers, allowing curl to expand. If too large, mist with water *lightly*.

TOOLS AND APPLIANCES REQUIRED
Towel
Wide-tooth comb
Quartz or diffusion dryer
Mist bottle
Spray shine (optional)
Hair spray (optional)

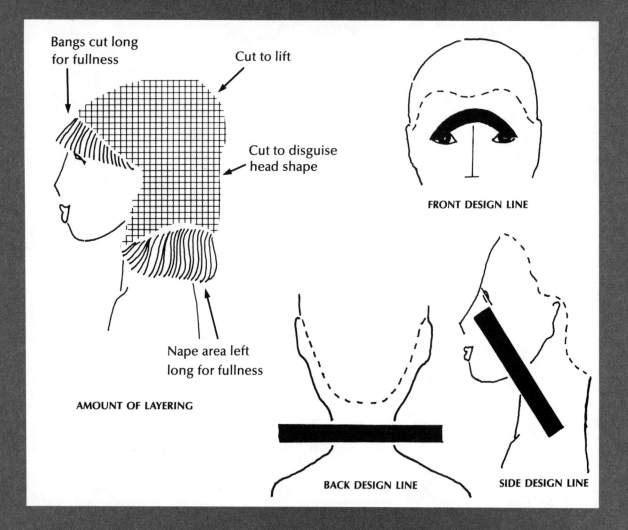

Bangs cut long for fullness

Cut to lift

Cut to disguise head shape

Nape area left long for fullness

AMOUNT OF LAYERING

FRONT DESIGN LINE

BACK DESIGN LINE

SIDE DESIGN LINE

THIS STYLE HIDES

Head shape
Head size
Profile
Low forehead
Front hairline
Nape hairline
Short neck
Hair condition

THIS STYLE HIGHLIGHTS

Ears
Face shape
Chin
Jawline
Hairline in front of ears

BODY PROPORTIONS

Suitable for medium, tall, and large proportions

THIS IS A *MINIMUM CARE* STYLE FOR CURLY HAIR.

THIS IS A *TEMPORARY* STYLE FOR STRAIGHT HAIR.

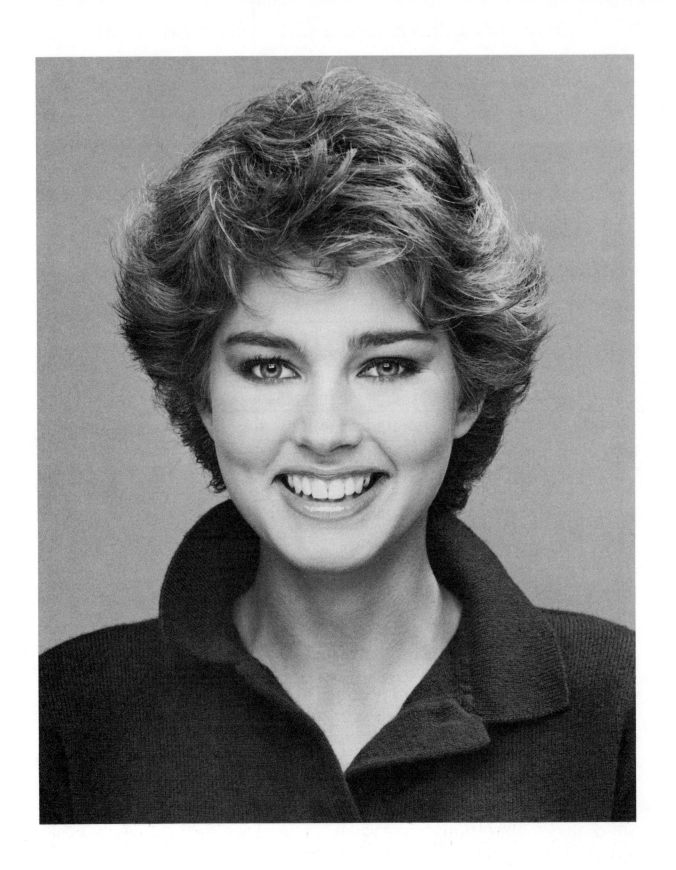

20 Short and sassy

Your Hair's Characteristics | Stylability

TEXTURE	FORMATION	QUANTITY	HAIR TYPE	CODE	TIMING*	SKILL RATING
FINE	STRAIGHT	THIN	1	WP4 ■	20 to 25 mins.	2 to 3
	STRAIGHT	MEDIUM	2	WP5 ■		
	STRAIGHT	THICK	3	WP6 ■		
	WAVY	THIN	4	C13 □		
	WAVY	MEDIUM	5	■		
	WAVY	THICK	6	■		
	CURLY	THIN	7	X		
	CURLY	MEDIUM	8	X		
	CURLY	THICK	9	X		
MEDIUM	STRAIGHT	THIN	10	WP13 ■	20 to 25 mins.	2 to 3
	STRAIGHT	MEDIUM	11	WP14 ■		
	STRAIGHT	THICK	12	WP15 ■		
	WAVY	THIN	13	C22 □		
	WAVY	MEDIUM	14	■		
	WAVY	THICK	15	■		
	CURLY	THIN	16	X		
	CURLY	MEDIUM	17	X		
	CURLY	THICK	18	X		
COARSE	STRAIGHT	THIN	19	WP22 ■	20 to 25 mins.	2 to 3
	STRAIGHT	MEDIUM	20	WP23 ■		
	STRAIGHT	THICK	21	WP24 ■		
	WAVY	THIN	22	C23 □		
	WAVY	MEDIUM	23	■		
	WAVY	THICK	24	■		
	CURLY	THIN	25	X		
	CURLY	MEDIUM	26	X		
	CURLY	THICK	27	X		

■ GOOD   □ POSSIBLE   X NOT RECOMMENDED

S STRAIGHTENING   **C** COLORING   **WP** WAVY PERM   **CP** CURLY PERM

*25% extra time for porous hair

Finishing and Styling Hints

SPECIAL TIPS

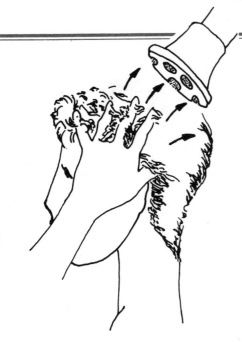

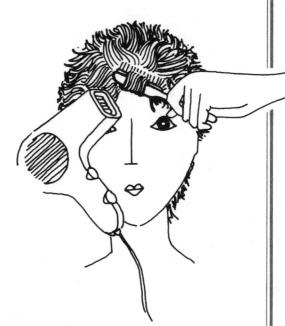

Towel dry to remove moisture, then dry with diffuser. Direct hair with fingers, drying roots and mid-lengths. Turn over ends with fingers to encourage wave.

If bangs or sides get untidy, turn them on a brush (vent or Denman). Apply warm heat from blow-dryer to tip ends casually.

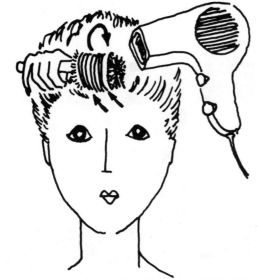

If bangs become too curly, stretch gently by using a large-diameter round brush and blow dryer. Try not to get a too perfect finish— allow your cut and wave to work together.

TOOLS AND APPLIANCES REQUIRED
Towel
Diffusion dryer
Denman and vent or round-bristle brush
Blow-dryer

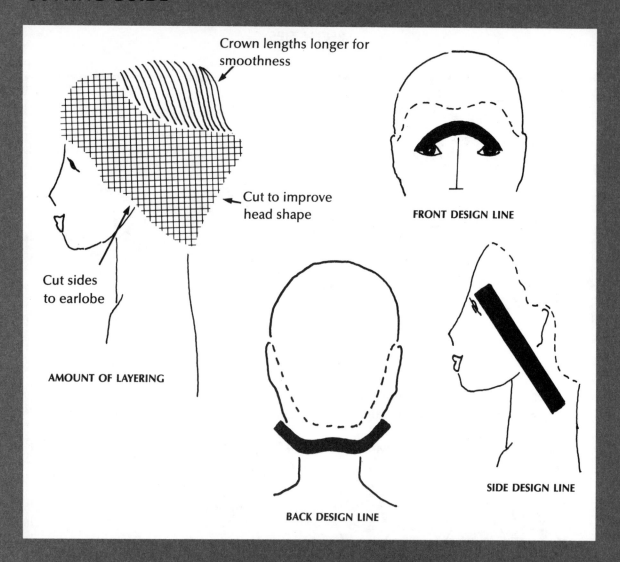

Crown lengths longer for smoothness

Cut to improve head shape

Cut sides to earlobe

AMOUNT OF LAYERING

FRONT DESIGN LINE

BACK DESIGN LINE

SIDE DESIGN LINE

THIS STYLE HIDES

Head shape
Head size
Profile
Ears
Receding Hairline
Low forehead
Narrow temples
Sparse hair at temples
Wide temples
Front hairline
Nape hairline
Hairline in front of ears

THIS STYLE HIGHLIGHTS

Face shape
Neck shapes: wide,
    short, long, thin
Hair condition

BODY PROPORTIONS

Suitable for petite,
small, medium,
and tall proportions

THIS IS A *MINIMUM CARE* STYLE FOR WAVY HAIR.

THIS IS A *TEMPORARY* STYLE FOR STRAIGHT HAIR.

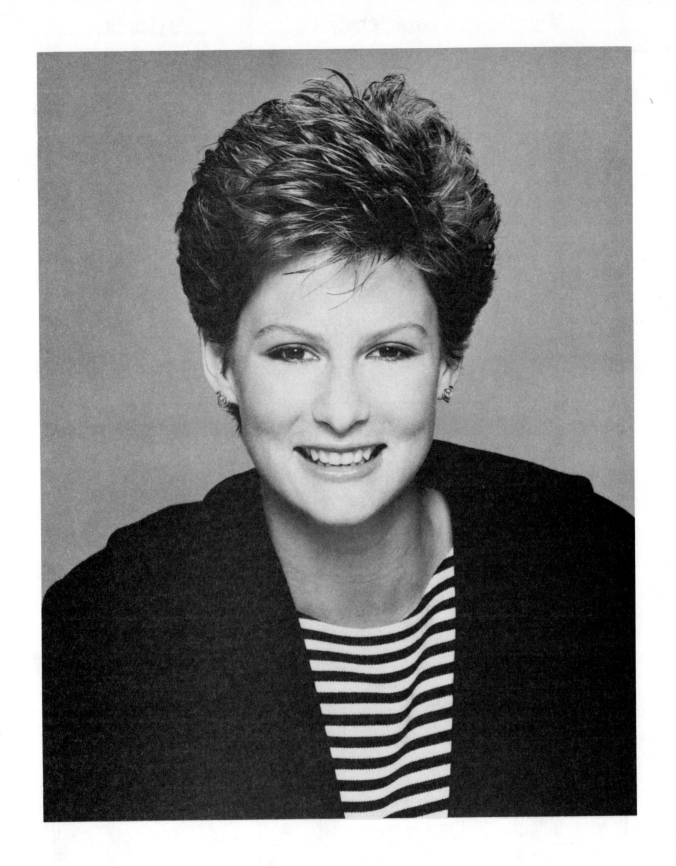

21 Short and chic

Your Hair's Characteristics | Stylability

TEXTURE	FORMATION		QUANTITY	HAIR TYPE	CODE	TIMING*	SKILL RATING
FINE	STRAIGHT		THIN	1	C10 ■		
			MEDIUM	2	■		
			THICK	3	■		
	WAVY		THIN	4	C13 ■	10 to 20 mins.	2 to 3
			MEDIUM	5	■		
			THICK	6	■		
	CURLY		THIN	7	X		
			MEDIUM	8	X		
			THICK	9	S3 ■		
MEDIUM	STRAIGHT		THIN	10	C19 ■		
			MEDIUM	11	■		
			THICK	12	■		
	WAVY		THIN	13	■	10 to 20 mins.	2 to 3
			MEDIUM	14	■		
			THICK	15	■		
	CURLY		THIN	16	S10 ■		
			MEDIUM	17	S11 ■		
			THICK	18	S12 ■		
COARSE	STRAIGHT		THIN	19	C20 ■		
			MEDIUM	20	■		
			THICK	21	■		
	WAVY		THIN	22	C23 ■	10 to 20 mins.	2 to 3
			MEDIUM	23	■		
			THICK	24	■		
	CURLY		THIN	25	S19 ■		
			MEDIUM	26	S20 ■		
			THICK	27	S21 ■		

172

■ GOOD   □ POSSIBLE   X NOT RECOMMENDED   S STRAIGHTENING   C COLORING   WP WAVY PERM   CP CURLY PERM

* 25% extra time for porous hair

Finishing and Styling Hints

SPECIAL TIPS

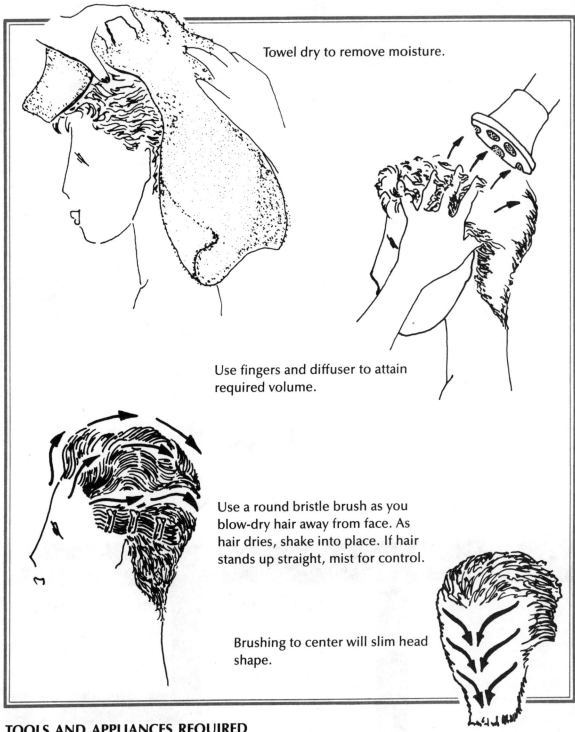

Towel dry to remove moisture.

Use fingers and diffuser to attain required volume.

Use a round bristle brush as you blow-dry hair away from face. As hair dries, shake into place. If hair stands up straight, mist for control.

Brushing to center will slim head shape.

TOOLS AND APPLIANCES REQUIRED
Towel
Vent or Denman brush
Quartz or diffusion dryer
Short clips
Mist bottle
Hair spray (optional)

CUTTING GUIDE

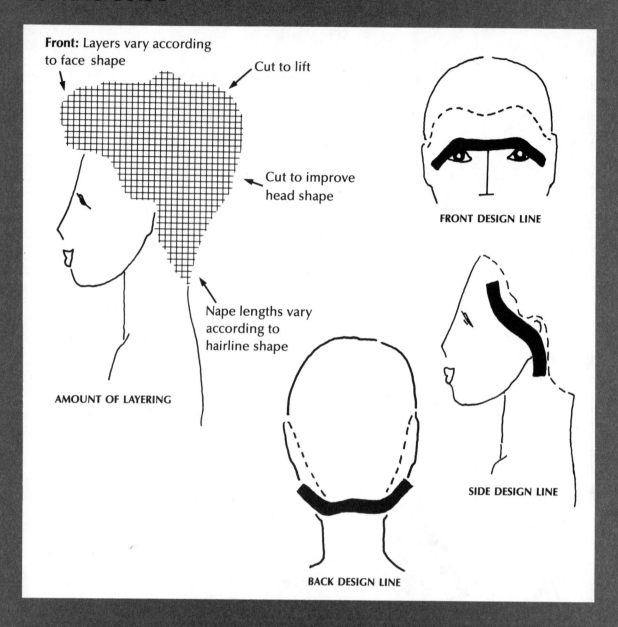

Front: Layers vary according to face shape

Cut to lift

Cut to improve head shape

Nape lengths vary according to hairline shape

AMOUNT OF LAYERING

FRONT DESIGN LINE

SIDE DESIGN LINE

BACK DESIGN LINE

THIS STYLE HIDES

Head shape
Head size
Profile
Receding hairline
Low forehead
Narrow temples
Sparse hair at temples
Wide temples
Front hairline

THIS STYLE HIGHLIGHTS

Ears
Face shape
Chin
Jawline
Nape hairline
Hairline in front of ears
Neck shape: wide, short, long, thin
Hair condition

BODY PROPORTIONS

Suitable for petite, small, and medium proportions

THIS IS A *MINIMUM CARE* STYLE FOR STRAIGHT AND WAVY HAIR.

174

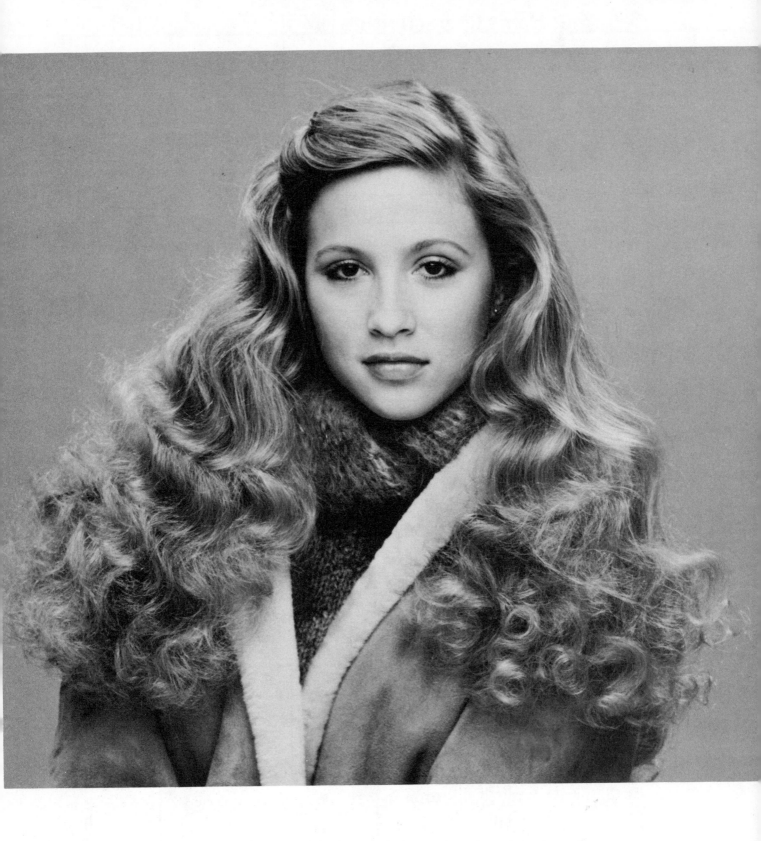

22 The long, lovely, natural look for healthy hair

Your Hair's Characteristics

Stylability

TEXTURE	FORMATION	QUANTITY	HAIR TYPE	CODE	TIMING*	SKILL RATING
FINE	STRAIGHT	THIN	1	X		
		MEDIUM	2	X		
		THICK	3	X		
	WAVY	THIN	4	C13 ■	35 to 55 mins.	4
		MEDIUM	5	■		
		THICK	6	■		
	CURLY	THIN	7	X		
		MEDIUM	8	X		
		THICK	9	X		
MEDIUM	STRAIGHT	THIN	10	X		
		MEDIUM	11	X		
		THICK	12	X		
	WAVY	THIN	13	C22 ■	35 to 55 mins.	4
		MEDIUM	14	■		
		THICK	15	■		
	CURLY	THIN	16	X		
		MEDIUM	17	X		
		THICK	18	X		
COARSE	STRAIGHT	THIN	19	X		
		MEDIUM	20	X		
		THICK	21	X		
	WAVY	THIN	22	C23 ■	35 to 55 mins.	4
		MEDIUM	23	■		
		THICK	24	■		
	CURLY	THIN	25	X		
		MEDIUM	26	X		
		THICK	27	X		

■ GOOD   ☐ POSSIBLE   X NOT RECOMMENDED   **S** STRAIGHTENING   **C** COLORING   **WP** WAVY PERM   **CP** CURLY PERM

176

* 25% extra time for porous hair

Finishing and Styling Hints

SPECIAL TIPS

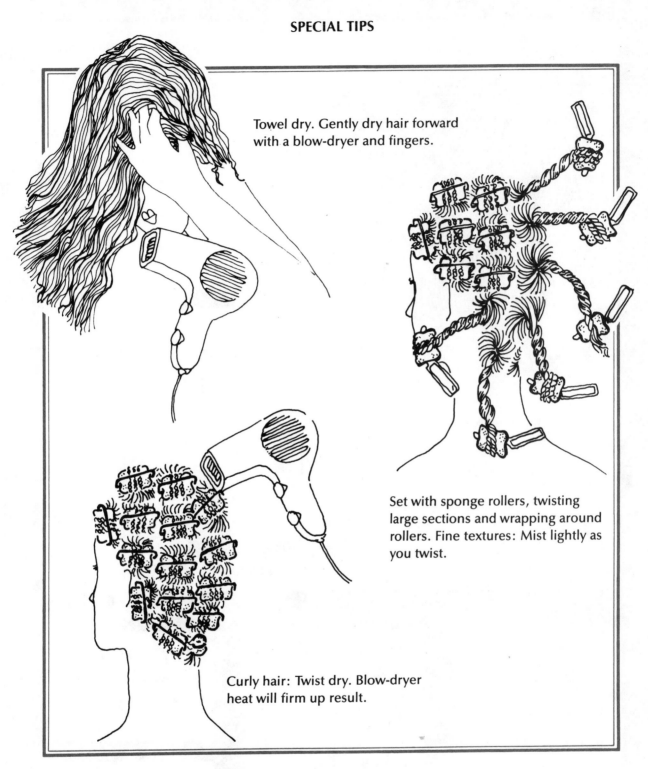

Towel dry. Gently dry hair forward with a blow-dryer and fingers.

Set with sponge rollers, twisting large sections and wrapping around rollers. Fine textures: Mist lightly as you twist.

Curly hair: Twist dry. Blow-dryer heat will firm up result.

TOOLS AND APPLIANCES REQUIRED

Towel
Wide-tooth comb
Rattail comb
Denman brush
Blow-dryer

Sponge rollers
Ribbon
Mist bottle (for fine textures)
Hair spray (optional)

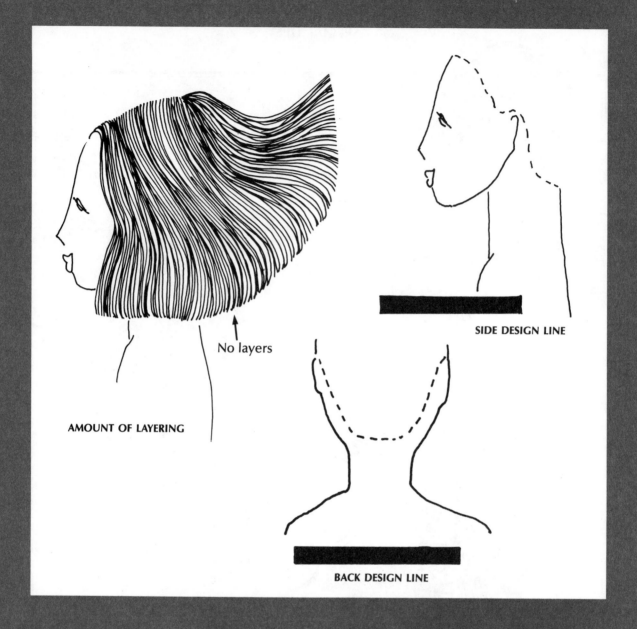

AMOUNT OF LAYERING

No layers

SIDE DESIGN LINE

BACK DESIGN LINE

THIS STYLE HIDES

Head shape
Head size
Profile
Ears
Wide face
Chin
Jawline
Nape hairline
Hairline in front of ears
Neck shapes: wide,
   short, long, thin

THIS STYLE HIGHLIGHTS

Thin face
Long face
Receding hairline
Low forehead
Narrow temples
Sparse hair at temples
Wide temples
Front hairline
Hair condition

BODY PROPORTIONS

Suitable for small,
medium, and tall
proportions

THIS IS A *MINIMUM CARE* STYLE FOR WAVY AND CURLY HAIR.

THIS IS A *TEMPORARY* STYLE FOR STRAIGHT HAIR.

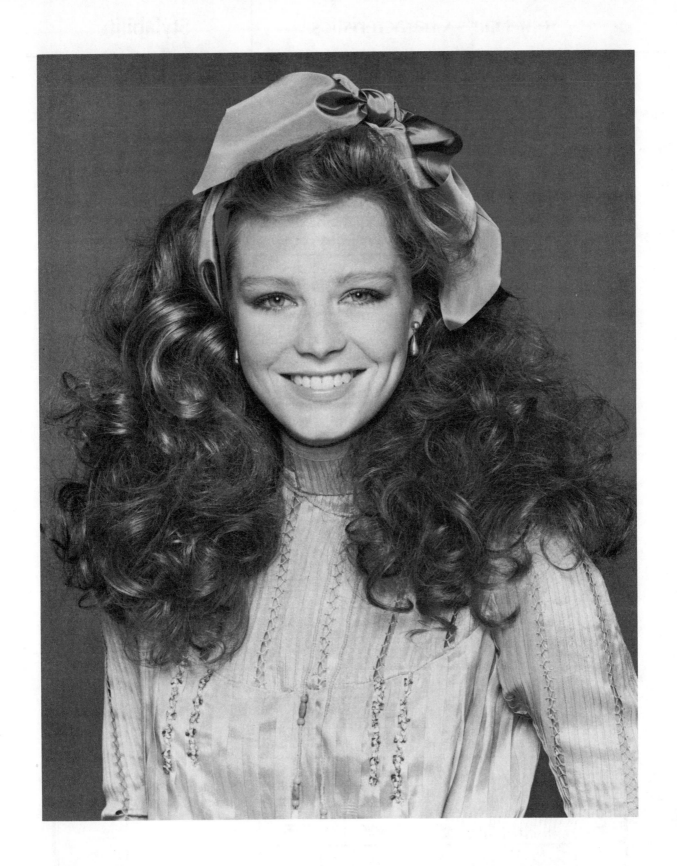

23 Innocent curl

Your Hair's Characteristics | Stylability

TEXTURE	FORMATION	QUANTITY	HAIR TYPE	CODE	TIMING*	SKILL RATING
FINE	STRAIGHT	THIN	1	WP4 ■	30 to 40 mins.	3 to 4
		MEDIUM	2	WP5 ■		
		THICK	3	WP6 ■		
	WAVY	THIN	4	C13 ■		
		MEDIUM	5	■		
		THICK	6	■		
	CURLY	THIN	7	C16 □		
		MEDIUM	8	□		
		THICK	9	□		
MEDIUM	STRAIGHT	THIN	10	WP13 ■	35 to 40 mins.	3 to 4
		MEDIUM	11	WP14 ■		
		THICK	12	WP15 ■		
	WAVY	THIN	13	C22 ■		
		MEDIUM	14	■		
		THICK	15	■		
	CURLY	THIN	16	C25 □		
		MEDIUM	17	□		
		THICK	18	□		
COARSE	STRAIGHT	THIN	19	WP22 ■	40 to 50 mins.	3 to 4
		MEDIUM	20	WP23 ■		
		THICK	21	WP24 ■		
	WAVY	THIN	22	C23 ■		
		MEDIUM	23	■		
		THICK	24	■		
	CURLY	THIN	25	C26 □		
		MEDIUM	26	□		
		THICK	27	□		

180

■ GOOD □ POSSIBLE X NOT RECOMMENDED S STRAIGHTENING C COLORING WP WAVY PERM CP CURLY PERM

* 25% extra time for porous hair

Finishing and Styling Hints

SPECIAL TIPS

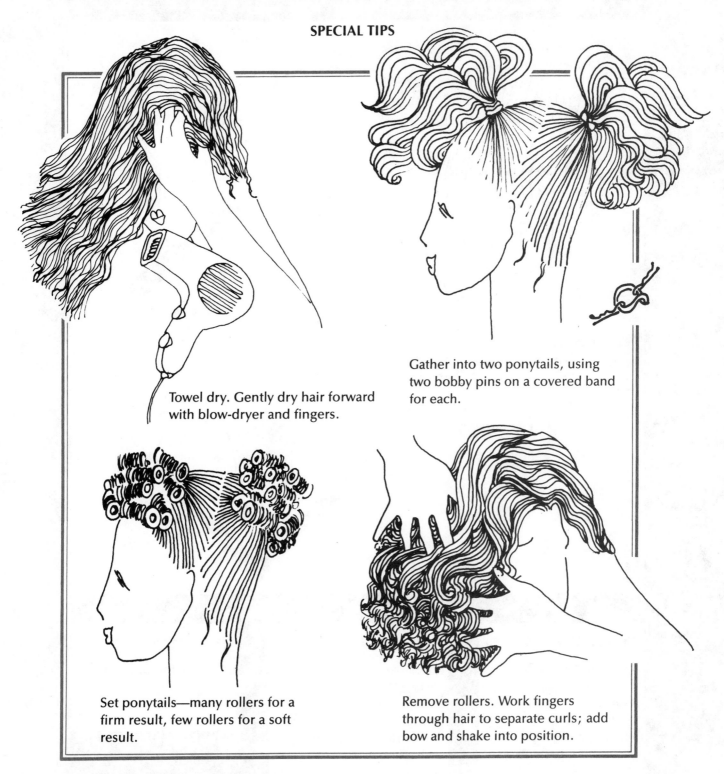

Towel dry. Gently dry hair forward with blow-dryer and fingers.

Gather into two ponytails, using two bobby pins on a covered band for each.

Set ponytails—many rollers for a firm result, few rollers for a soft result.

Remove rollers. Work fingers through hair to separate curls; add bow and shake into position.

TOOLS AND APPLIANCES REQUIRED

Towel
Wide-tooth comb
Rattail comb
Denman or vent brush
Blow-dryer

Hot rollers
Covered bands with bobby pins
Ribbon
Hair spray (optional)
Antistatic material (for fine textures)

CUTTING GUIDE

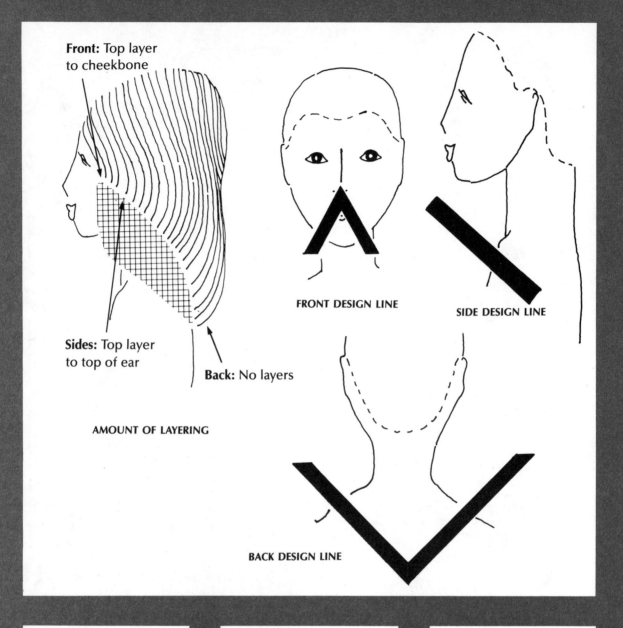

Front: Top layer to cheekbone

Sides: Top layer to top of ear

Back: No layers

AMOUNT OF LAYERING

FRONT DESIGN LINE

SIDE DESIGN LINE

BACK DESIGN LINE

THIS STYLE HIDES

Head shape
Head size
Profile
Nape hairline
Neck shapes: wide,
   short, long, thin

THIS STYLE HIGHLIGHTS

Ears
Face Shape
Chin
Jawline
All hairlines except nape
   hairline
Hair condition

BODY PROPORTIONS

Suitable for medium,
tall, and large
proportions

THIS IS A *MINIMUM CARE* STYLE FOR WAVY-TO-CURLY HAIR.

THIS IS A *TEMPORARY* STYLE FOR STRAIGHT HAIR.

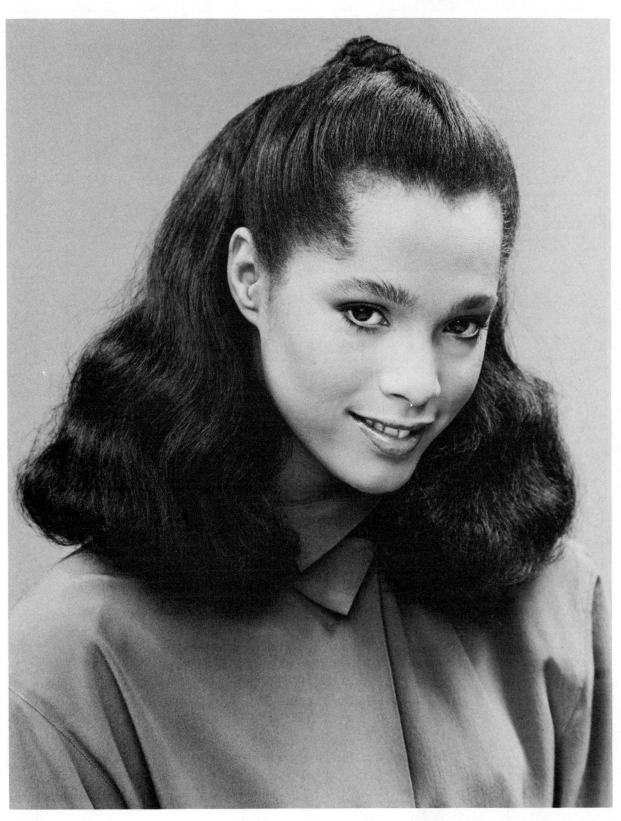

24 Braid and bob

Your Hair's Characteristics | Stylability

TEXTURE	FORMATION	QUANTITY	HAIR TYPE	CODE	TIMING	SKILL RATING
FINE	STRAIGHT	THIN	1	■	**Note:** This style does not require freshly shampooed hair. Time estimates are for dry-hair styling. 15 to 20 mins.	3
FINE	STRAIGHT	MEDIUM	2	■		
FINE	STRAIGHT	THICK	3	■		
FINE	WAVY	THIN	4	■		
FINE	WAVY	MEDIUM	5	■		
FINE	WAVY	THICK	6	■		
FINE	CURLY	THIN	7	■		
FINE	CURLY	MEDIUM	8	■		
FINE	CURLY	THICK	9	■		
MEDIUM	STRAIGHT	THIN	10	■	15 to 20 mins.	3
MEDIUM	STRAIGHT	MEDIUM	11	■		
MEDIUM	STRAIGHT	THICK	12	■		
MEDIUM	WAVY	THIN	13	■		
MEDIUM	WAVY	MEDIUM	14	■		
MEDIUM	WAVY	THICK	15	■		
MEDIUM	CURLY	THIN	16	■		
MEDIUM	CURLY	MEDIUM	17	■		
MEDIUM	CURLY	THICK	18	■		
COARSE	STRAIGHT	THIN	19	■	15 to 20 mins.	3
COARSE	STRAIGHT	MEDIUM	20	■		
COARSE	STRAIGHT	THICK	21	■		
COARSE	WAVY	THIN	22	■		
COARSE	WAVY	MEDIUM	23	■		
COARSE	WAVY	THICK	24	■		
COARSE	CURLY	THIN	25	■		
COARSE	CURLY	MEDIUM	26	■		
COARSE	CURLY	THICK	27	■		

184

■ GOOD   □ POSSIBLE   X NOT RECOMMENDED   S STRAIGHTENING   C COLORING   WP WAVY PERM   CP CURLY PERM

Finishing and Styling Hints

SPECIAL TIPS

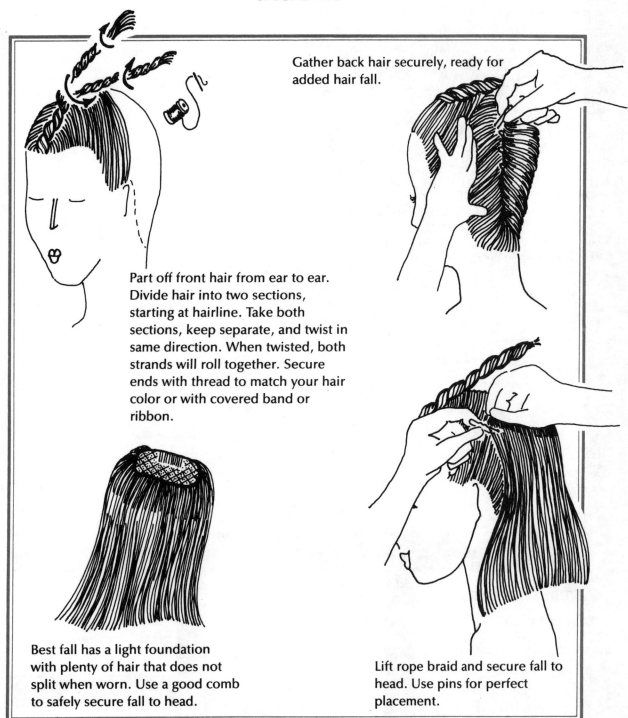

Gather back hair securely, ready for added hair fall.

Part off front hair from ear to ear. Divide hair into two sections, starting at hairline. Take both sections, keep separate, and twist in same direction. When twisted, both strands will roll together. Secure ends with thread to match your hair color or with covered band or ribbon.

Best fall has a light foundation with plenty of hair that does not split when worn. Use a good comb to safely secure fall to head.

Lift rope braid and secure fall to head. Use pins for perfect placement.

TOOLS AND APPLIANCES REQUIRED

Wide-tooth comb
Denman or vent brush
Flat-back brush
Bobby pins
Hairpins

Needle and thread
Fall (synthetic fiber okay)
Ribbon (optional)
Hair spray (optional)

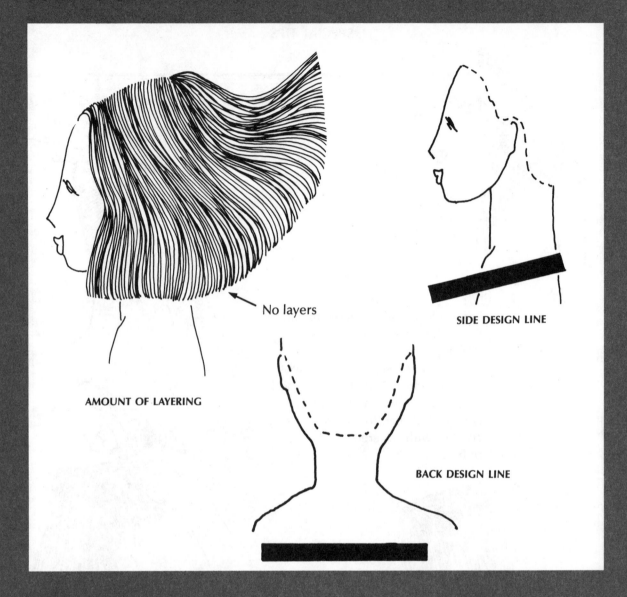

No layers

AMOUNT OF LAYERING

SIDE DESIGN LINE

BACK DESIGN LINE

THIS STYLE HIDES

Head shape
Head size
Profile
Nape hairline
Neck shapes: wide,
    short, long, thin
Hair condition

THIS STYLE HIGHLIGHTS

Ears
Face shape
Receding hairline
Low forehead
Narrow temples
Sparse hair at temples
Wide temples
Front hairline
Hairline in front of ears

BODY PROPORTIONS

Suitable for petite,
small, medium,
and tall proportions

THIS IS A *MINIMUM CARE* STYLE FOR ALL FORMATIONS.

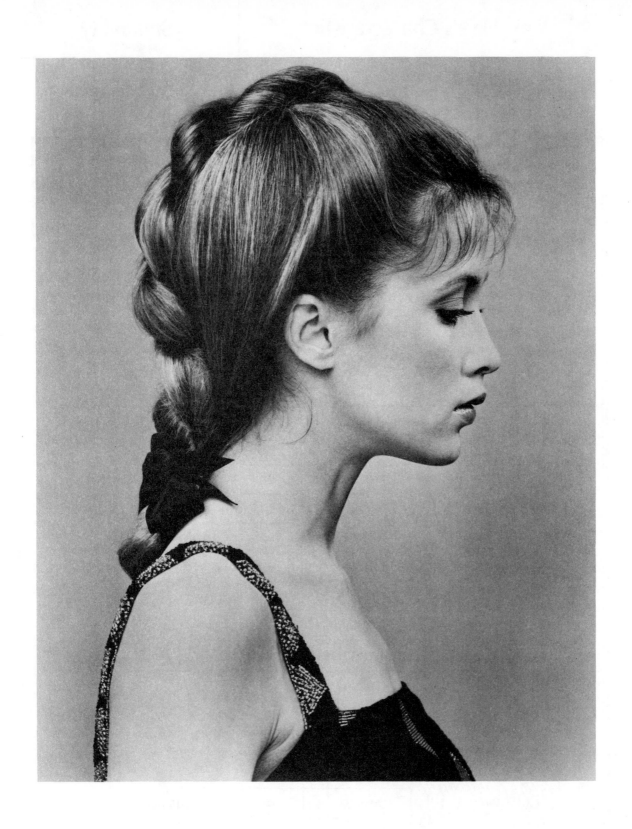

25 Divine twine

Your Hair's Characteristics   Stylability

TEXTURE	FORMATION	QUANTITY	HAIR TYPE	CODE	TIMING	SKILL RATING
FINE	STRAIGHT	THIN	1	□	**Note:** This style does not require freshly shampooed hair. Time estimates are for dry-hair styling.	
	STRAIGHT	MEDIUM	2	■		
	STRAIGHT	THICK	3	■		
	WAVY	THIN	4	□		
	WAVY	MEDIUM	5	■		
	WAVY	THICK	6	■		
	CURLY	THIN	7	□	10 to 15 mins.	3
	CURLY	MEDIUM	8	■		
	CURLY	THICK	9	■		
MEDIUM	STRAIGHT	THIN	10	□		
	STRAIGHT	MEDIUM	11	■		
	STRAIGHT	THICK	12	■		
	WAVY	THIN	13	□		
	WAVY	MEDIUM	14	■	10 to 15 mins.	3
	WAVY	THICK	15	■		
	CURLY	THIN	16	□		
	CURLY	MEDIUM	17	■		
	CURLY	THICK	18	■		
COARSE	STRAIGHT	THIN	19	□		
	STRAIGHT	MEDIUM	20	■		
	STRAIGHT	THICK	21	■		
	WAVY	THIN	22	□		
	WAVY	MEDIUM	23	■	10 to 15 mins.	3
	WAVY	THICK	24	■		
	CURLY	THIN	25	□		
	CURLY	MEDIUM	26	■		
	CURLY	THICK	27	■		

■ GOOD   □ POSSIBLE   X NOT RECOMMENDED   **S** STRAIGHTENING   **C** COLORING   **WP** WAVY PERM   **CP** CURLY PERM

Finishing and Styling Hints

SPECIAL TIPS

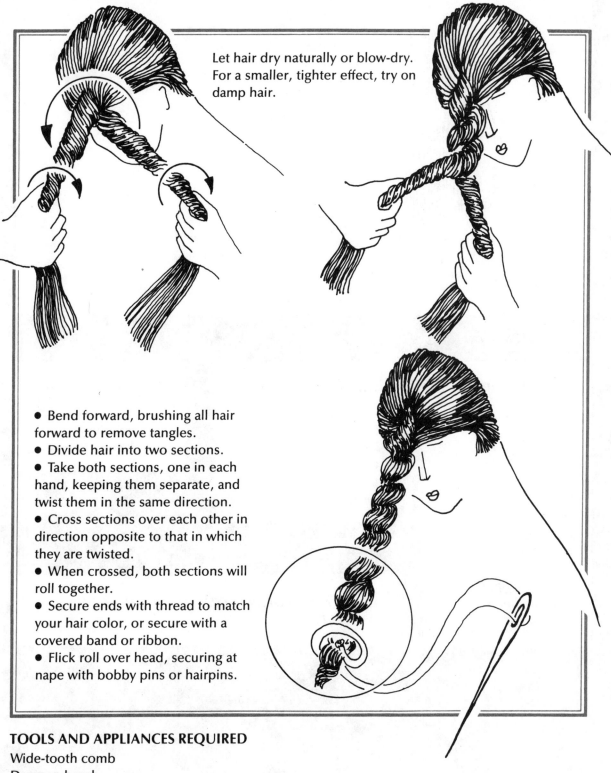

Let hair dry naturally or blow-dry. For a smaller, tighter effect, try on damp hair.

- Bend forward, brushing all hair forward to remove tangles.
- Divide hair into two sections.
- Take both sections, one in each hand, keeping them separate, and twist them in the same direction.
- Cross sections over each other in direction opposite to that in which they are twisted.
- When crossed, both sections will roll together.
- Secure ends with thread to match your hair color, or secure with a covered band or ribbon.
- Flick roll over head, securing at nape with bobby pins or hairpins.

TOOLS AND APPLIANCES REQUIRED

Wide-tooth comb
Denman brush
Mist bottle
Bobby pins
Hairpins
Needle and thread
Ribbon

CUTTING GUIDE

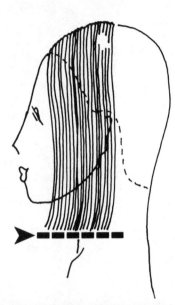

MINIMUM LENGTH REQUIRED

Top length at least below chin

THIS STYLE HIDES

Head shape
Profile
Receding hairline
Low forehead
Narrow temples
Sparse hair at temples
Wide temples
Front hairline
Nape hairline
Neck shapes: wide,
    short, long, thin
Hair condition
Bad haircut

THIS STYLE HIGHLIGHTS

Head size
Ears
Face Shape
Chin
Jawline
All hairlines

BODY PROPORTIONS

Suitable for petite,
small, medium,
and tall proportions

THIS IS A *TEMPORARY* STYLE BUT *MINIMUM CARE* WHEN STYLED INTO PLACE.

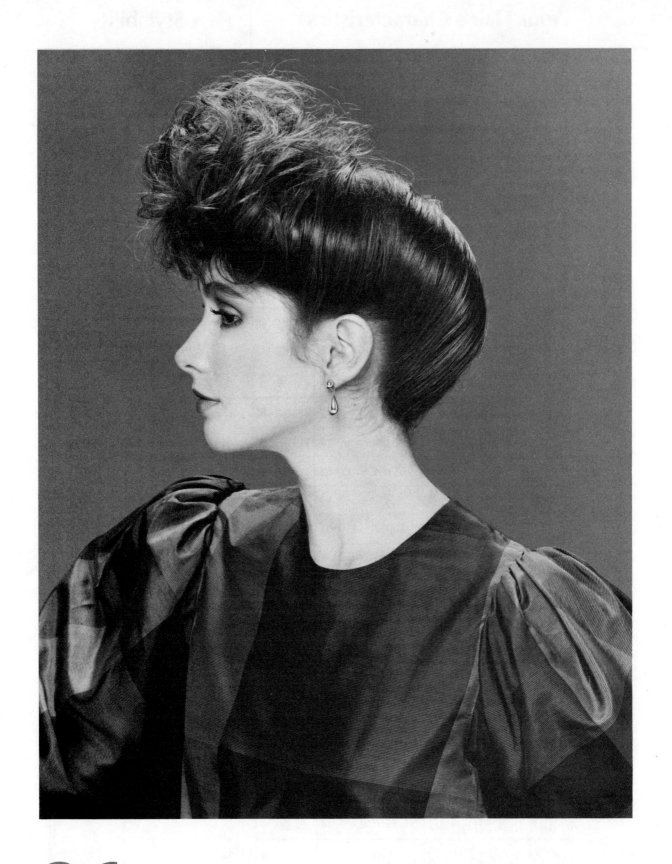

26 The modern look for evening

Your Hair's Characteristics — Stylability

TEXTURE	FORMATION	QUANTITY	HAIR TYPE	CODE	TIMING*	SKILL RATING
FINE	STRAIGHT	THIN	1	WP4 ■	**Note:** This style does not require freshly shampooed hair. Time estimates are for dry-hair styling.	3 to 4
FINE	STRAIGHT	MEDIUM	2	WP5 ■		
FINE	STRAIGHT	THICK	3	WP6 ■		
FINE	WAVY	THIN	4	C13 ■		
FINE	WAVY	MEDIUM	5	■		
FINE	WAVY	THICK	6	■		
FINE	CURLY	THIN	7	C16 ■	15 to 25 mins.	
FINE	CURLY	MEDIUM	8	■		
FINE	CURLY	THICK	9	■		
MEDIUM	STRAIGHT	THIN	10	WP13 ■		3 to 4
MEDIUM	STRAIGHT	MEDIUM	11	WP14 ■		
MEDIUM	STRAIGHT	THICK	12	WP15 ■		
MEDIUM	WAVY	THIN	13	C22 ■		
MEDIUM	WAVY	MEDIUM	14	■	15 to 25 mins.	
MEDIUM	WAVY	THICK	15	■		
MEDIUM	CURLY	THIN	16	C25 ■		
MEDIUM	CURLY	MEDIUM	17	■		
MEDIUM	CURLY	THICK	18	■		
COARSE	STRAIGHT	THIN	19	WP22 ■		3 to 4
COARSE	STRAIGHT	MEDIUM	20	WP23 ■		
COARSE	STRAIGHT	THICK	21	WP24 ■		
COARSE	WAVY	THIN	22	C23 ■		
COARSE	WAVY	MEDIUM	23	■	15 to 25 mins.	
COARSE	WAVY	THICK	24	■		
COARSE	CURLY	THIN	25	C26 ■		
COARSE	CURLY	MEDIUM	26	■		
COARSE	CURLY	THICK	27	■		

■ GOOD   ☐ POSSIBLE   X NOT RECOMMENDED   S STRAIGHTENING   C COLORING   **WP** WAVY PERM   **CP** CURLY PERM

Finishing and Styling Hints

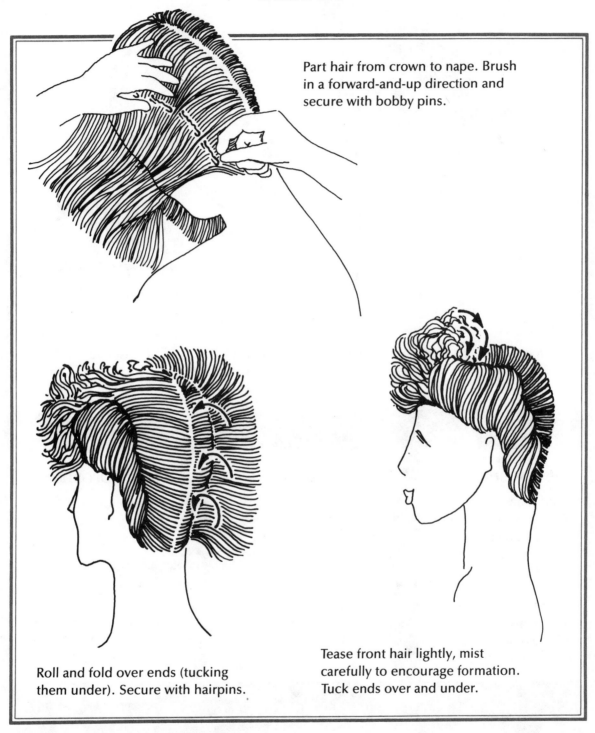

Part hair from crown to nape. Brush in a forward-and-up direction and secure with bobby pins.

Roll and fold over ends (tucking them under). Secure with hairpins.

Tease front hair lightly, mist carefully to encourage formation. Tuck ends over and under.

TOOLS AND APPLIANCES REQUIRED

Wide-tooth comb	Hairpins
Rattail comb	Flat-back brush
Mist bottle	Hair spray (optional)
Bobby pins	Long clips (optional)

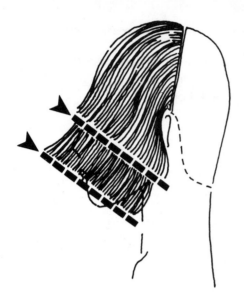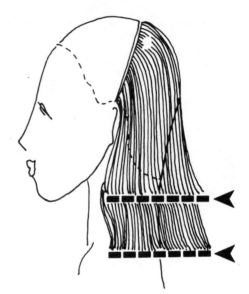

MINIMUM LENGTHS REQUIRED

Front: Top layers at least over brow. Bottom lengths at least below nose.

Back: Top layer at least over hairline. Bottom length at least to shoulder.

THIS STYLE HIDES

Head shape
Head size
Receding hairline
Low forehead
Narrow temples
Sparse hair at temples
Wide temples
Front hairline
Bad haircut
Hair condition

THIS STYLE HIGHLIGHTS

Ears
Face shape
Chin
Jawline
Profile
Nape hairline
Neck shapes: wide,
    short, long, thin
Hairline in front of ears

BODY PROPORTIONS

Suitable for small, medium, and tall proportions

THIS IS A *TEMPORARY* STYLE FOR ALL FORMATIONS.

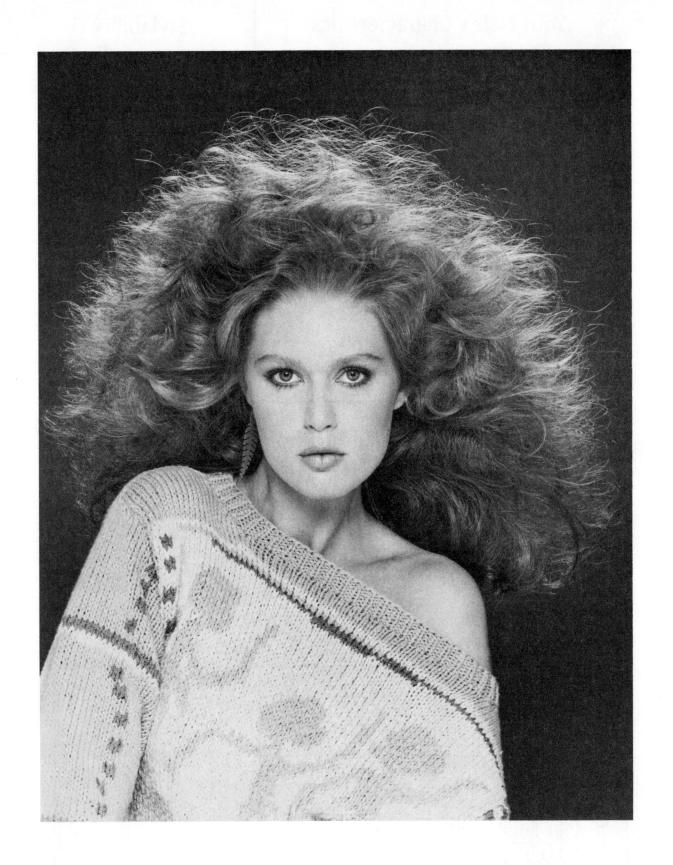

27 Razzzz!

Your Hair's Characteristics | Stylability

TEXTURE	FORMATION	QUANTITY	HAIR TYPE	CODE		TIMING*	SKILL RATING
FINE	STRAIGHT	THIN	1	WP4	☐		
		MEDIUM	2	WP5	☐		
		THICK	3	WP6	☐		
	WAVY	THIN	4	C13	☐	40 to 50 mins.	3 to 4
		MEDIUM	5		☐		
		THICK	6		☐		
	CURLY	THIN	7	C16	■		
		MEDIUM	8		■		
		THICK	9		■		
MEDIUM	STRAIGHT	THIN	10	CP16	■		
		MEDIUM	11	CP17	■		
		THICK	12	CP18	■		
	WAVY	THIN	13	C22	☐	40 to 50 mins.	3 to 4
		MEDIUM	14		☐		
		THICK	15		☐		
	CURLY	THIN	16	C25	■		
		MEDIUM	17		■		
		THICK	18		■		
COARSE	STRAIGHT	THIN	19	WP22	☐		
		MEDIUM	20	WP23	☐		
		THICK	21	WP24	☐		
	WAVY	THIN	22	C23	☐	40 to 50 mins.	3 to 4
		MEDIUM	23		☐		
		THICK	24		☐		
	CURLY	THIN	25		■		
		MEDIUM	26		■		
		THICK	27		■		

■ GOOD   ☐ POSSIBLE   X NOT RECOMMENDED   S STRAIGHTENING   C COLORING   WP WAVY PERM   CP CURLY PERM

*25 % extra time for porous hair

Finishing and Styling Hints

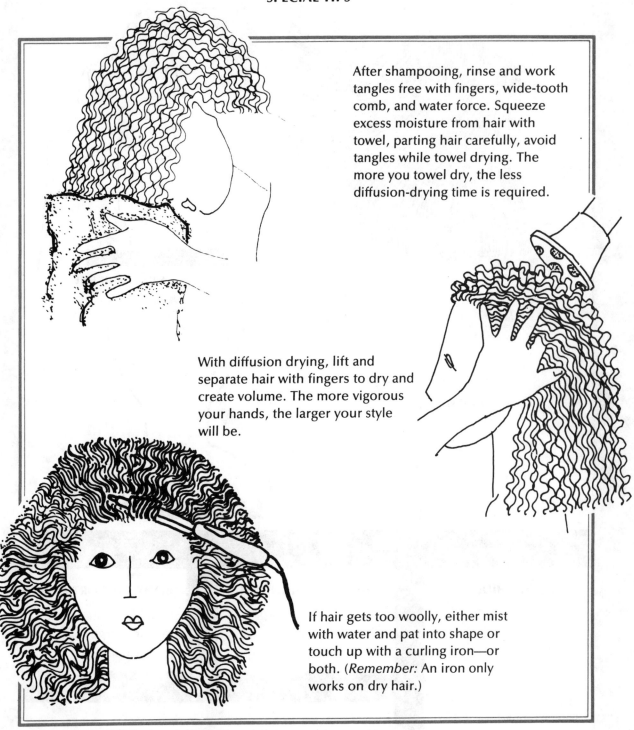

After shampooing, rinse and work tangles free with fingers, wide-tooth comb, and water force. Squeeze excess moisture from hair with towel, parting hair carefully, avoid tangles while towel drying. The more you towel dry, the less diffusion-drying time is required.

With diffusion drying, lift and separate hair with fingers to dry and create volume. The more vigorous your hands, the larger your style will be.

If hair gets too woolly, either mist with water and pat into shape or touch up with a curling iron—or both. (*Remember:* An iron only works on dry hair.)

TOOLS AND APPLIANCES REQUIRED
Towel
Wide-tooth comb
Diffusion dryer
Small- or large-diameter curling iron (small diameter makes curls; large diameter smooths and waves)
Spray shine or hairdressing, such as Vitapointe (optional)

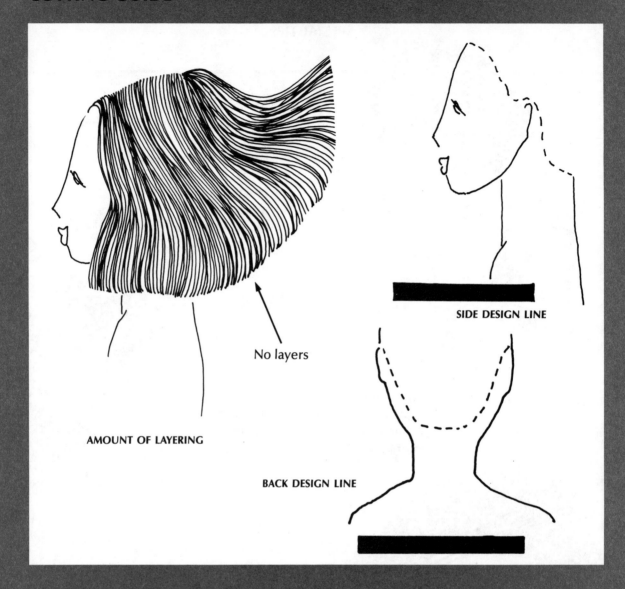

No layers

AMOUNT OF LAYERING

SIDE DESIGN LINE

BACK DESIGN LINE

THIS STYLE HIDES

Head shape
Head size
Profile
Ears
Chin
Jawline
Low forehead
Narrow temples
Sparse hair at temples
Wide temples
Front hairline
Nape hairline
Hairline in front of ears
Neck shapes
Hair condition

THIS STYLE HIGHLIGHTS

Face shape
Receding hairline

BODY PROPORTIONS

Suitable for medium, tall, and large proportions

THIS IS A *MINIMUM CARE* STYLE FOR CURLY AND WAVY HAIR.

THIS IS A *TEMPORARY* STYLE FOR STRAIGHT HAIR.

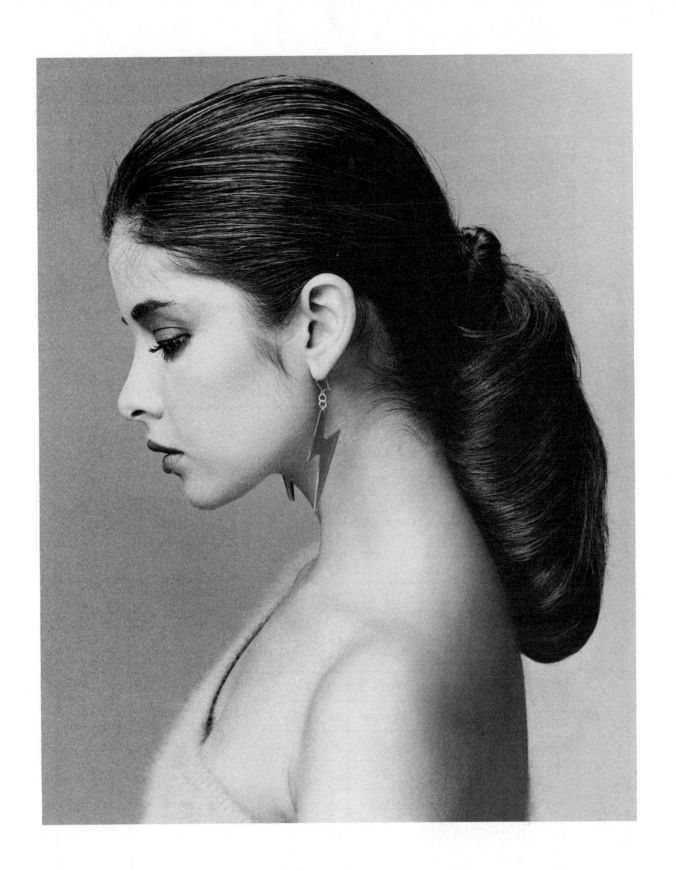

28 Subtle and soft for day or night

Your Hair's Characteristics | Stylability

TEXTURE	FORMATION	QUANTITY	HAIR TYPE	CODE	TIMING	SKILL RATING
FINE	STRAIGHT	THIN	1	■	**Note:** This style does not require freshly shampooed hair. Time estimates are for dry-hair styling. 5 to 10 mins.	1 to 3
FINE	STRAIGHT	MEDIUM	2	■		
FINE	STRAIGHT	THICK	3	■		
FINE	WAVY	THIN	4	■		
FINE	WAVY	MEDIUM	5	■		
FINE	WAVY	THICK	6	■		
FINE	CURLY	THIN	7	■		
FINE	CURLY	MEDIUM	8	■		
FINE	CURLY	THICK	9	■		
MEDIUM	STRAIGHT	THIN	10	■	5 to 10 mins.	1 to 3
MEDIUM	STRAIGHT	MEDIUM	11	■		
MEDIUM	STRAIGHT	THICK	12	■		
MEDIUM	WAVY	THIN	13	■		
MEDIUM	WAVY	MEDIUM	14	■		
MEDIUM	WAVY	THICK	15	■		
MEDIUM	CURLY	THIN	16	■		
MEDIUM	CURLY	MEDIUM	17	■		
MEDIUM	CURLY	THICK	18	■		
COARSE	STRAIGHT	THIN	19	■	5 to 10 mins.	1 to 3
COARSE	STRAIGHT	MEDIUM	20	■		
COARSE	STRAIGHT	THICK	21	■		
COARSE	WAVY	THIN	22	■		
COARSE	WAVY	MEDIUM	23	■		
COARSE	WAVY	THICK	24	■		
COARSE	CURLY	THIN	25	■		
COARSE	CURLY	MEDIUM	26	■		
COARSE	CURLY	THICK	27	■		

■ GOOD   ☐ POSSIBLE   X NOT RECOMMENDED   **S** STRAIGHTENING   **C** COLORING   **WP** WAVY PERM   **CP** CURLY PERM

SPECIAL TIPS

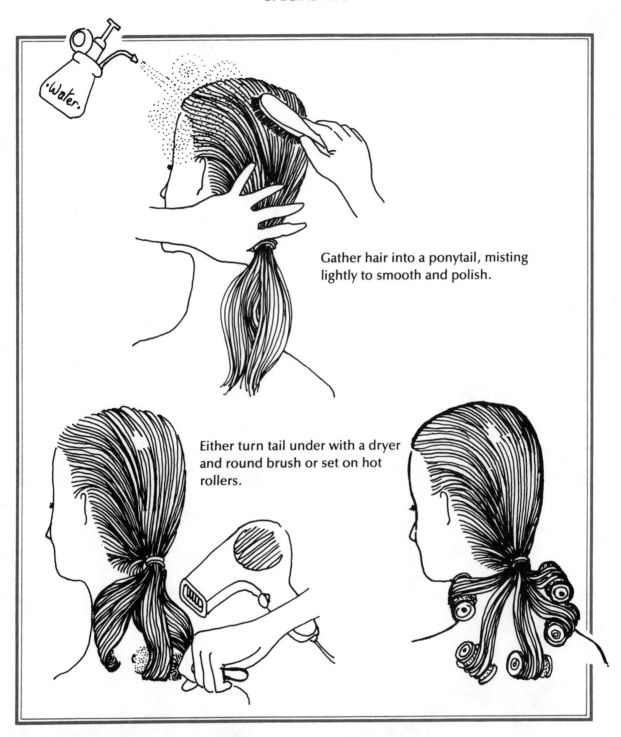

Gather hair into a ponytail, misting lightly to smooth and polish.

Either turn tail under with a dryer and round brush or set on hot rollers.

TOOLS AND APPLIANCES REQUIRED

Flat-back brush
Wide-tooth comb
Rattail comb
Round brush and dryer
Hot rollers
Mist bottle
Covered band

201

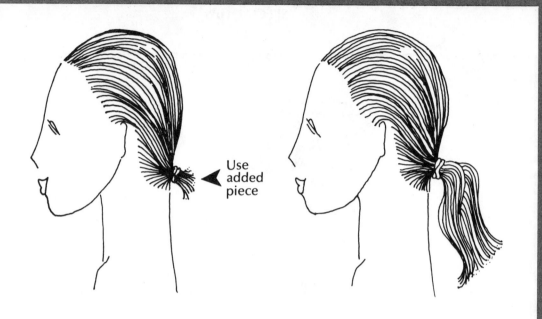

► Use added piece

MINIMUM LENGTH REQUIRED

Long enough to gather into a ponytail at nape. The shorter the hair, the higher the tail.

Or, if the tail reaches your shoulder when gathered, the thicker your hair, the bigger the tail; the thinner your hair, the smaller the tail.

THIS STYLE HIDES

Nape hairline
Neck shapes: wide, short, long, thin

THIS STYLE HIGHLIGHTS

Head shape
Head size
Profile
Ears
Face shape
Chin
Jawline
All hairlines except nape hairline
Hair condition

BODY PROPORTIONS

Suitable for petite, small, medium, and tall proportions

THIS IS A *MINIMUM CARE* STYLE FOR ALL FORMATIONS.

29

Fabulously folded

Your Hair's Characteristics

Stylability

TEXTURE	FORMATION		QUANTITY	HAIR TYPE	CODE	TIMING	SKILL RATING
FINE	STRAIGHT		THIN	1	C10 ☐	**Note:** This style does not require freshly shampooed hair. Time estimates are for dry-hair styling. 20 to 30 mins.	3 to 5
			MEDIUM	2	C11 ☐		
			THICK	3	C12 ☐		
	WAVY		THIN	4	C13 ■		
			MEDIUM	5	■		
			THICK	6	■		
	CURLY		THIN	7	C16 ■		
			MEDIUM	8	■		
			THICK	9	■		
MEDIUM	STRAIGHT		THIN	10	C19 ☐	20 to 30 mins.	3 to 5
			MEDIUM	11	C20 ☐		
			THICK	12	C21 ☐		
	WAVY		THIN	13	C22 ■		
			MEDIUM	14	■		
			THICK	15	■		
	CURLY		THIN	16	C25 ■		
			MEDIUM	17	■		
			THICK	18	■		
COARSE	STRAIGHT		THIN	19	☐	20 to 30 mins.	3 to 5
			MEDIUM	20	☐		
			THICK	21	☐		
	WAVY		THIN	22	■		
			MEDIUM	23	■		
			THICK	24	■		
	CURLY		THIN	25	C26 ■		
			MEDIUM	26	■		
			THICK	27	■		

■ GOOD ☐ POSSIBLE X NOT RECOMMENDED   **S** STRAIGHTENING **C** COLORING **WP** WAVY PERM **CP** CURLY PERM

Finishing and Styling Hints

SPECIAL TIPS

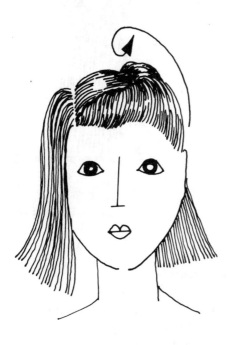

This can be done on wet or dry hair.
● Make a side parting.
● Part from ear to ear.
● Smooth down all hair. Remove tangles.
● Twist front over in a roll and secure with barrette. Repeat on other side.

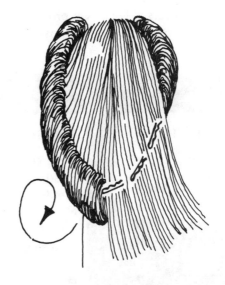

● Brush down back hair. Secure firmly at nape with a row of bobby pins.
● Roll over one side and fasten in place with bobby pins and hairpins. Repeat on opposite side.
● Complete style by tucking in center back section.

Mist hair continually with water to keep wispy ends in place. . . . Or use initial light misting of spray. Be sure pins are well anchored in hair.

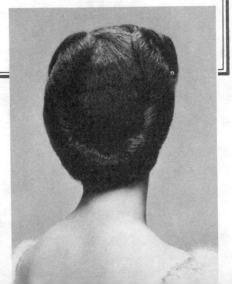

TOOLS AND APPLIANCES REQUIRED

Rattail comb
Long clips
Bobby pins
Hairpins
Flat-back brush
Mist bottle
Hair spray

BACK VIEW

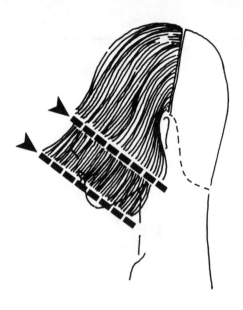 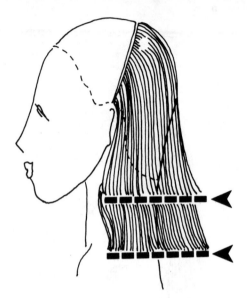

MINIMUM LENGTHS REQUIRED

Front: Top layers at least over brow. Bottom lengths at least below nose.

Back: Top layer at least over hairline. Bottom length at least to shoulder.

THIS STYLE HIDES

Hair condition
Bad haircut

THIS STYLE HIGHLIGHTS

Head shape
Head size
Profile
Nose
Ears
Face shape
Chin
Jawline
All hairlines
Neck shapes: wide,
  short, long, thin

BODY PROPORTIONS

Suitable for petite, small, and medium proportions

THIS IS A *MINIMUM CARE* STYLE FOR ALL FORMATIONS WHEN STYLED INTO PLACE.

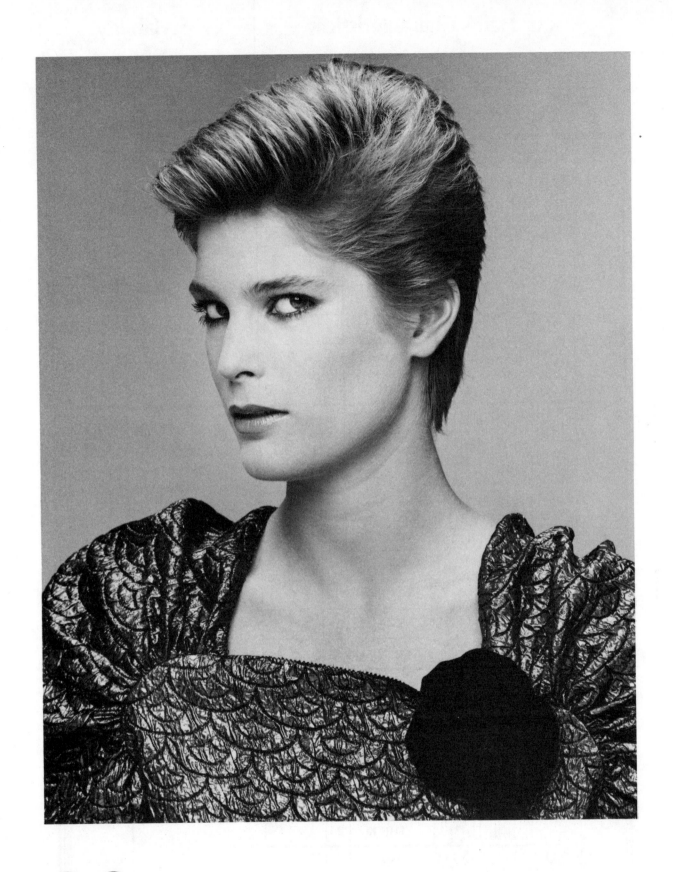

30 Short sophistication

Your Hair's Characteristics | Stylability

TEXTURE	FORMATION	QUANTITY	HAIR TYPE	CODE	TIMING*	SKILL RATING
FINE	STRAIGHT	THIN	1	C10 ■	5 to 10 mins.	2 to 3
		MEDIUM	2	■		
		THICK	3	■		
	WAVY	THIN	4	C13 □		
		MEDIUM	5	□		
		THICK	6	□		
	CURLY	THIN	7	X		
		MEDIUM	8	X		
		THICK	9	S3 ■		
MEDIUM	STRAIGHT	THIN	10	C19 ■	10 to 15 mins.	2 to 3
		MEDIUM	11	■		
		THICK	12	■		
	WAVY	THIN	13	C22 □		
		MEDIUM	14	□		
		THICK	15	□		
	CURLY	THIN	16	S10 ■		
		MEDIUM	17	S11 ■		
		THICK	18	S12 ■		
COARSE	STRAIGHT	THIN	19	C20 ■	10 to 15 mins.	2 to 3
		MEDIUM	20	■		
		THICK	21	■		
	WAVY	THIN	22	C23 □		
		MEDIUM	23	□		
		THICK	24	□		
	CURLY	THIN	25	S19 ■		
		MEDIUM	26	S20 ■		
		THICK	27	S21 ■		

■ GOOD □ POSSIBLE X NOT RECOMMENDED S STRAIGHTENING C COLORING WP WAVY PERM CP CURLY PERM

208

*25% extra time for porous hair

Finishing and Styling Hints

SPECIAL TIPS

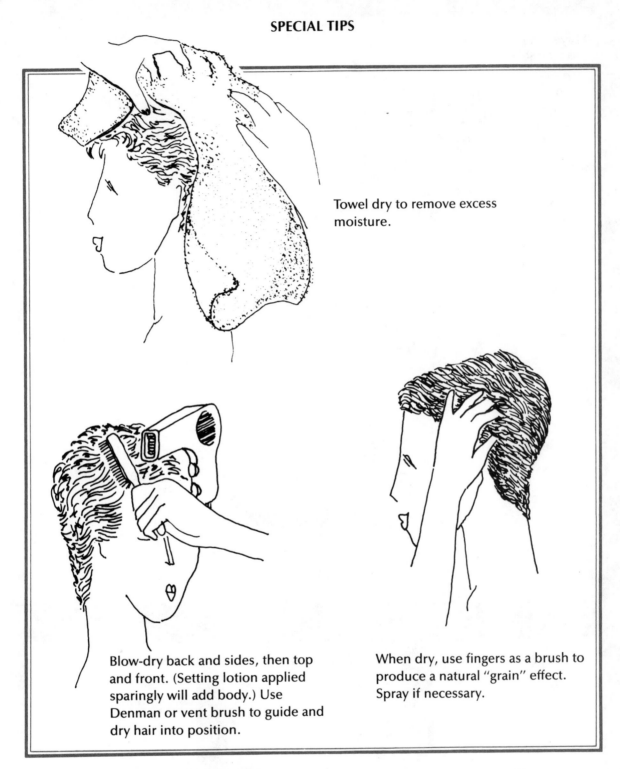

Towel dry to remove excess moisture.

Blow-dry back and sides, then top and front. (Setting lotion applied sparingly will add body.) Use Denman or vent brush to guide and dry hair into position.

When dry, use fingers as a brush to produce a natural "grain" effect. Spray if necessary.

TOOLS AND APPLIANCES REQUIRED
Towel
Denman or vent brush
Blow-dryer
Liquid setting lotion (optional)
Hair spray (optional)
Antistatic material (for fine textures)

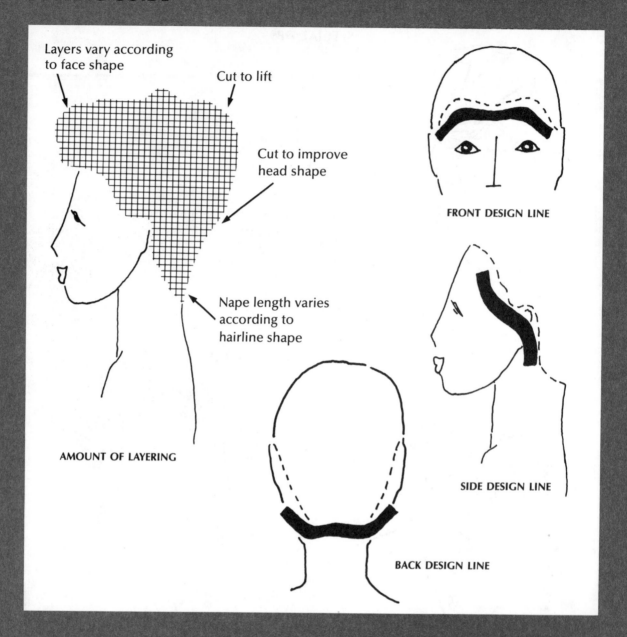

Layers vary according to face shape

Cut to lift

Cut to improve head shape

Nape length varies according to hairline shape

AMOUNT OF LAYERING

FRONT DESIGN LINE

SIDE DESIGN LINE

BACK DESIGN LINE

THIS STYLE HIDES

Profile
Head shape

THIS STYLE HIGHLIGHTS

Nose
Jawline
Chin
Ears
Neck

BODY PROPORTIONS

Not suitable for large proportions

THIS IS A *MINIMUM CARE* STYLE FOR STRAIGHT HAIR.
THIS IS A *TEMPORARY* STYLE FOR WAVY-TO-CURLY HAIR.

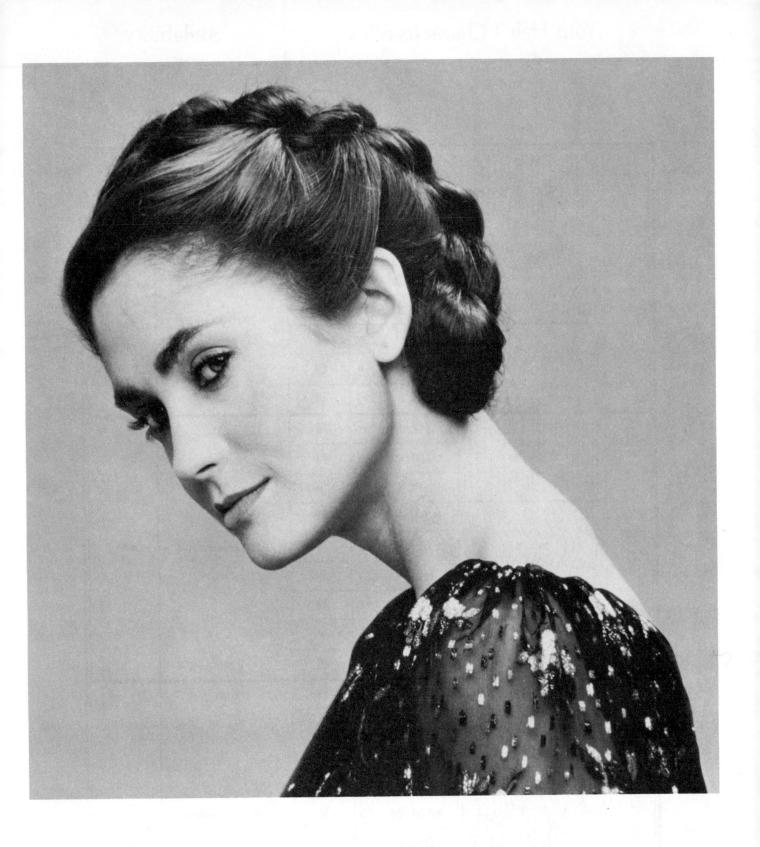

31 Gala braid

Your Hair's Characteristics | Stylability

TEXTURE	FORMATION	QUANTITY	HAIR TYPE	CODE	TIMING	SKILL RATING
FINE	STRAIGHT	THIN	1	■	**Note:** This style does not require freshly shampooed hair. Time estimates are for dry-hair styling. 20 to 30 mins.	4 to 5
FINE	STRAIGHT	MEDIUM	2	■		
FINE	STRAIGHT	THICK	3	■		
FINE	WAVY	THIN	4	■		
FINE	WAVY	MEDIUM	5	■		
FINE	WAVY	THICK	6	■		
FINE	CURLY	THIN	7	■		
FINE	CURLY	MEDIUM	8	■		
FINE	CURLY	THICK	9	■		
MEDIUM	STRAIGHT	THIN	10	■	20 to 30 mins.	4 to 5
MEDIUM	STRAIGHT	MEDIUM	11	■		
MEDIUM	STRAIGHT	THICK	12	■		
MEDIUM	WAVY	THIN	13	■		
MEDIUM	WAVY	MEDIUM	14	■		
MEDIUM	WAVY	THICK	15	■		
MEDIUM	CURLY	THIN	16	■		
MEDIUM	CURLY	MEDIUM	17	■		
MEDIUM	CURLY	THICK	18	■		
COARSE	STRAIGHT	THIN	19	■	20 to 30 mins.	4 to 5
COARSE	STRAIGHT	MEDIUM	20	■		
COARSE	STRAIGHT	THICK	21	■		
COARSE	WAVY	THIN	22	■		
COARSE	WAVY	MEDIUM	23	■		
COARSE	WAVY	THICK	24	■		
COARSE	CURLY	THIN	25	■		
COARSE	CURLY	MEDIUM	26	■		
COARSE	CURLY	THICK	27	■		

■ GOOD ☐ POSSIBLE **X** NOT RECOMMENDED   **S** STRAIGHTENING **C** COLORING **WP** WAVY PERM **CP** CURLY PERM

Finishing and Styling Hints

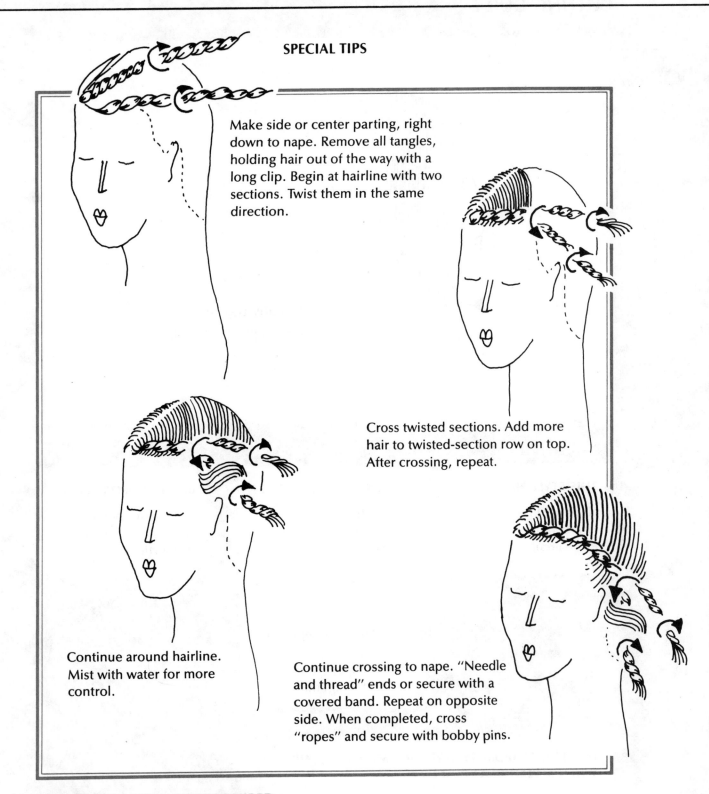

SPECIAL TIPS

Make side or center parting, right down to nape. Remove all tangles, holding hair out of the way with a long clip. Begin at hairline with two sections. Twist them in the same direction.

Cross twisted sections. Add more hair to twisted-section row on top. After crossing, repeat.

Continue around hairline. Mist with water for more control.

Continue crossing to nape. "Needle and thread" ends or secure with a covered band. Repeat on opposite side. When completed, cross "ropes" and secure with bobby pins.

TOOLS AND APPLIANCES REQUIRED

Pick	Small-diameter round brush
Wide-tooth comb	Bobby pins
Rattail comb	Human-hair hairnet or needle and thread
Flat-back or Denman brush	Spray shine (optional)
Long clips	Hair spray (optional)

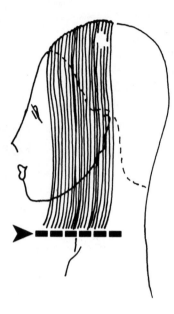

MINIMUM LENGTH REQUIRED

Top length at least below chin

THIS STYLE HIDES

Nape hairline
Hair condition
Bad haircut

THIS STYLE HIGHLIGHTS

Head shape
Head size
Profile
Ears
Face shape
Chin
Jawline
All hairlines except nape
  hairline
Neck shapes: wide,
  short, long, thin

BODY PROPORTIONS

Suitable for petite,
small, and medium
proportions

**THIS IS A *TEMPORARY* STYLE BUT *MINIMUM CARE*
WHEN STYLED INTO PLACE.**

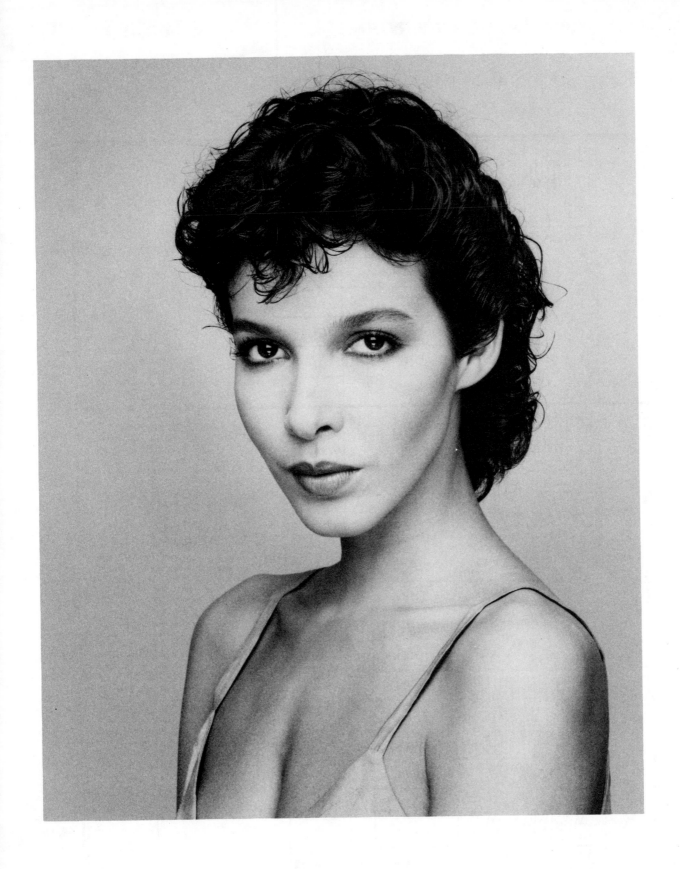

32 Short, easy-care waves

Your Hair's Characteristics | Stylability

TEXTURE	FORMATION	QUANTITY	HAIR TYPE	CODE	TIMING*	SKILL RATING
FINE	STRAIGHT	THIN	1	WP4 ■	25 to 30 mins.	2 to 3
FINE	STRAIGHT	MEDIUM	2	WP5 ■		
FINE	STRAIGHT	THICK	3	WP6 ■		
FINE	WAVY	THIN	4	C13 ■		
FINE	WAVY	MEDIUM	5	■		
FINE	WAVY	THICK	6	■		
FINE	CURLY	THIN	7	C16 ■		
FINE	CURLY	MEDIUM	8	■		
FINE	CURLY	THICK	9	■		
MEDIUM	STRAIGHT	THIN	10	WP13 ■	25 to 30 mins.	2 to 3
MEDIUM	STRAIGHT	MEDIUM	11	WP14 ■		
MEDIUM	STRAIGHT	THICK	12	WP15 ■		
MEDIUM	WAVY	THIN	13	C22 ■		
MEDIUM	WAVY	MEDIUM	14	■		
MEDIUM	WAVY	THICK	15	■		
MEDIUM	CURLY	THIN	16	C25 ■		
MEDIUM	CURLY	MEDIUM	17	■		
MEDIUM	CURLY	THICK	18	■		
COARSE	STRAIGHT	THIN	19	WP22 ■	25 to 30 mins.	2 to 3
COARSE	STRAIGHT	MEDIUM	20	WP23 ■		
COARSE	STRAIGHT	THICK	21	WP24 ■		
COARSE	WAVY	THIN	22	C23 ■		
COARSE	WAVY	MEDIUM	23	■		
COARSE	WAVY	THICK	24	■		
COARSE	CURLY	THIN	25	C26 ■		
COARSE	CURLY	MEDIUM	26	■		
COARSE	CURLY	THICK	27	■		

■ GOOD   ☐ POSSIBLE   X NOT RECOMMENDED   S STRAIGHTENING   C COLORING   WP WAVY PERM   CP CURLY PERM

216

*25% extra time for porous hair

Finishing and Styling Hints

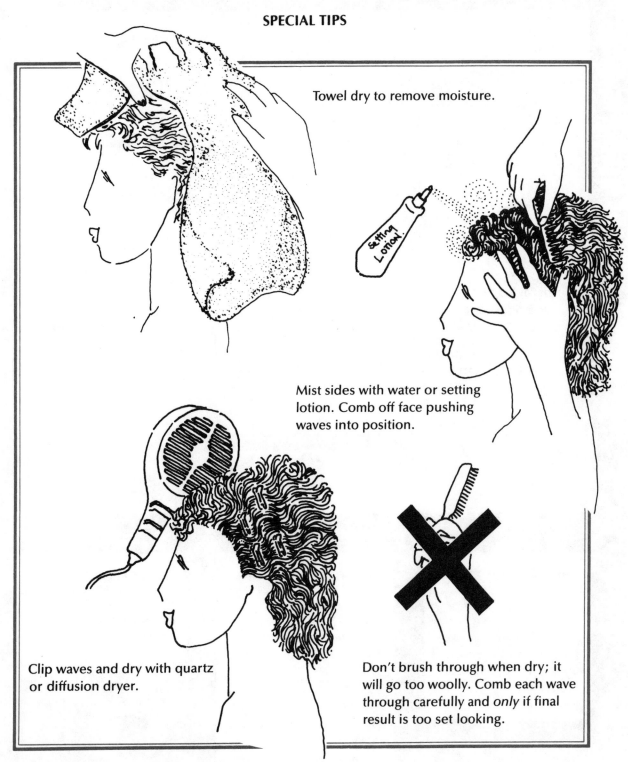

Towel dry to remove moisture.

Mist sides with water or setting lotion. Comb off face pushing waves into position.

Clip waves and dry with quartz or diffusion dryer.

Don't brush through when dry; it will go too woolly. Comb each wave through carefully and *only* if final result is too set looking.

TOOLS AND APPLIANCES REQUIRED
Towel
Wide-tooth comb
Quartz or diffusion dryer
Short clips
Mist bottle or setting lotion

CUTTING GUIDE

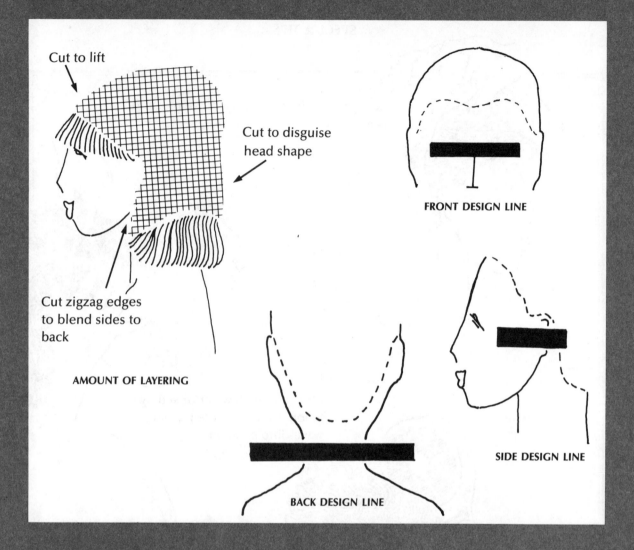

Cut to lift

Cut to disguise
head shape

Cut zigzag edges
to blend sides to
back

AMOUNT OF LAYERING

FRONT DESIGN LINE

BACK DESIGN LINE

SIDE DESIGN LINE

THIS STYLE HIDES

Head shape
Profile
Low forehead
Narrow temples
Sparse hair at temples
Front hairline
Nape hairline

THIS STYLE HIGHLIGHTS

Head size
Ears
Face shape
Chin
Jawline
Receding hairline
Wide temples
Hairline in front of ears
Neck shapes: wide,
    short, long, thin
Hair condition

BODY PROPORTIONS

Suitable for petite,
small, and medium
proportions.

THIS IS A *MINIMUM CARE* STYLE FOR WAVY AND CURLY HAIR.

THIS IS A *TEMPORARY* STYLE FOR STRAIGHT HAIR.

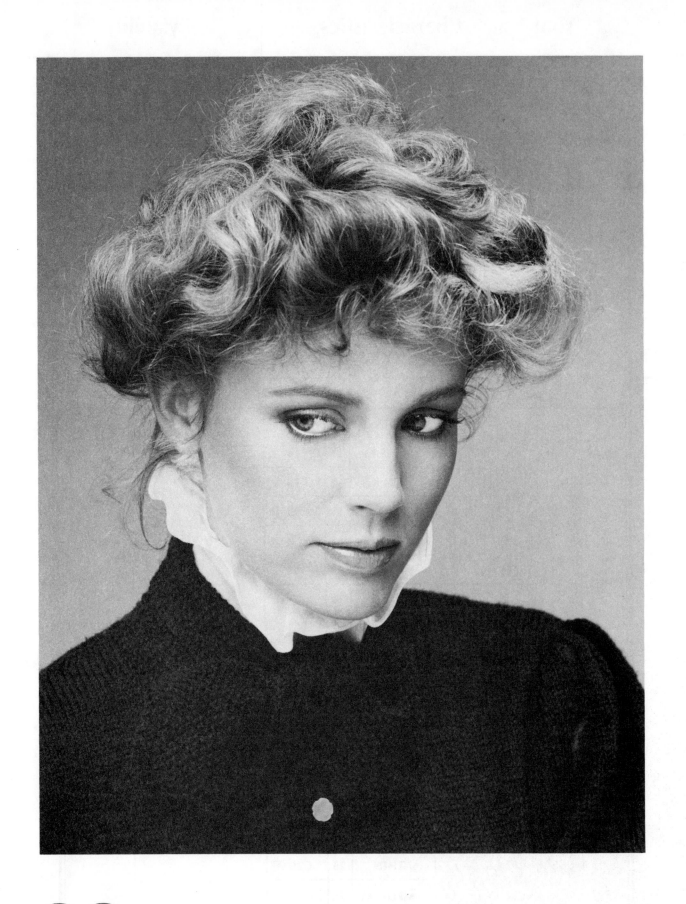

33 Informal elegance for fine hair

Your Hair's Characteristics | Stylability

TEXTURE	FORMATION	QUANTITY	HAIR TYPE	CODE	TIMING	SKILL RATING
FINE	STRAIGHT	THIN	1	WP4 ■	**Note:** Time estimates are for dry-hair styling.	3 to 4
		MEDIUM	2	WP5 ■		
		THICK	3	WP6 ■		
	WAVY	THIN	4	C13 ■		
		MEDIUM	5	■	10 to 20 mins.	
		THICK	6	■		
	CURLY	THIN	7	C16 ■		
		MEDIUM	8	■		
		THICK	9	■		
MEDIUM	STRAIGHT	THIN	10	WP13 ■		3
		MEDIUM	11	WP14 ■		
		THICK	12	WP15 ■		
	WAVY	THIN	13	C22 ■		
		MEDIUM	14	■	10 to 20 mins.	
		THICK	15	■		
	CURLY	THIN	16	C25 ■		
		MEDIUM	17	■		
		THICK	18	■		
COARSE	STRAIGHT	THIN	19	WP22 ■		3
		MEDIUM	20	WP23 ■		
		THICK	21	WP24 ■		
	WAVY	THIN	22	C23 ■		
		MEDIUM	23	■	10 to 20 mins.	
		THICK	24	■		
	CURLY	THIN	25	C26 ■		
		MEDIUM	26	■		
		THICK	27	■		

■ GOOD   □ POSSIBLE   X NOT RECOMMENDED   **S** STRAIGHTENING   **C** COLORING   **WP** WAVY PERM   **CP** CURLY PERM

Finishing and Styling Hints

SPECIAL TIPS

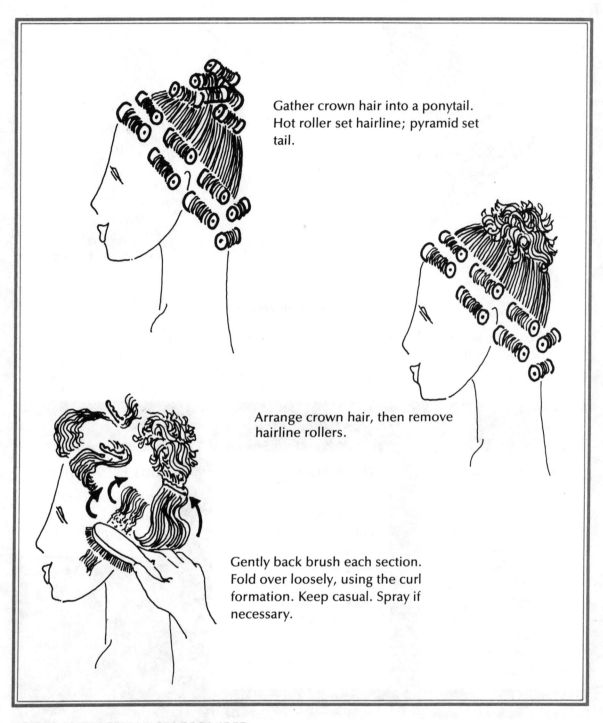

Gather crown hair into a ponytail. Hot roller set hairline; pyramid set tail.

Arrange crown hair, then remove hairline rollers.

Gently back brush each section. Fold over loosely, using the curl formation. Keep casual. Spray if necessary.

TOOLS AND APPLIANCES REQUIRED

Wide-tooth comb

Rattail comb	Covered band (or covered band with bobby pins)
Hot rollers	Flat-back brush
Bobby pins	Long clips (optional)
Hairpins	Hair spray (optional)

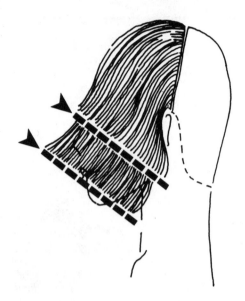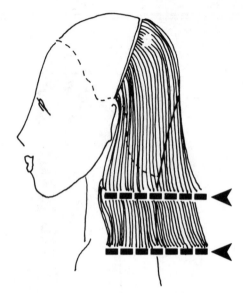

MINIMUM LENGTHS REQUIRED

Front: Top layers at least over brow. Bottom lengths at least below nose.

Back: Top layer at least over hairline. Bottom length at least to shoulder.

THIS STYLE HIDES

Head shape
Head size
Profile
Receding hairline
Low forehead
Narrow temples
Sparse hair at temples
Wide temples
Front hairline
Hair condition
Bad haircut

THIS STYLE HIGHLIGHTS

Ears
Face shape
Chin
Jawline
Nape hairline
Hairline in front of ears
Neck shapes: wide,
    short, long, thin

BODY PROPORTIONS

Suitable for petite, small, medium, and tall proportions

THIS IS A *MINIMUM CARE* STYLE FOR WAVY AND CURLY HAIR WHEN STYLED INTO PLACE.

THIS IS A *TEMPORARY* STYLE FOR STRAIGHT HAIR.

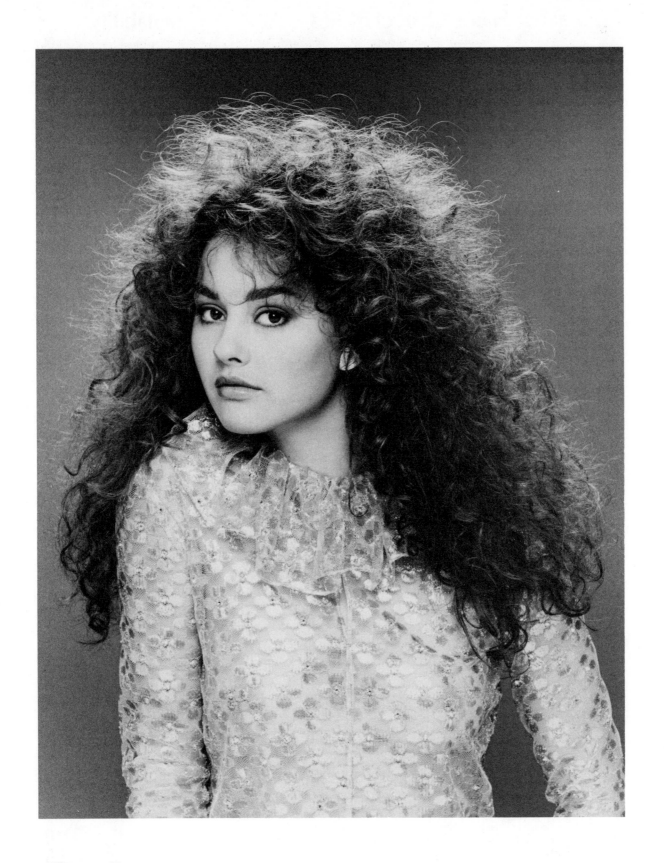

34
Sexy and sensual for curly hair

Your Hair's Characteristics | Stylability

TEXTURE	FORMATION	QUANTITY	HAIR TYPE	CODE	TIMING*	SKILL RATING
FINE	STRAIGHT	THIN	1	WP4 ☐	30 to 40 mins.	3 to 4
	STRAIGHT	MEDIUM	2	WP5 ☐		
	STRAIGHT	THICK	3	WP6 ☐		
	WAVY	THIN	4	C13 ☐		
	WAVY	MEDIUM	5	C14 ☐		
	WAVY	THICK	6	☐		
	CURLY	THIN	7	C16 ■		
	CURLY	MEDIUM	8	■		
	CURLY	THICK	9	■		
MEDIUM	STRAIGHT	THIN	10	CP16 ■	30 to 40 mins.	3 to 4
	STRAIGHT	MEDIUM	11	CP17 ■		
	STRAIGHT	THICK	12	CP18 ■		
	WAVY	THIN	13	C22 ☐		
	WAVY	MEDIUM	14	☐		
	WAVY	THICK	15	☐		
	CURLY	THIN	16	C25 ■		
	CURLY	MEDIUM	17	■		
	CURLY	THICK	18	■		
COARSE	STRAIGHT	THIN	19	WP22 ☐	30 to 40 mins.	3 to 4
	STRAIGHT	MEDIUM	20	WP23 ☐		
	STRAIGHT	THICK	21	WP24 ☐		
	WAVY	THIN	22	C23 ☐		
	WAVY	MEDIUM	23	☐		
	WAVY	THICK	24	☐		
	CURLY	THIN	25	C26 ■		
	CURLY	MEDIUM	26	■		
	CURLY	THICK	27	■		

■ GOOD   ☐ POSSIBLE   X NOT RECOMMENDED

S STRAIGHTENING   C COLORING   WP WAVY PERM   CP CURLY PERM

*25% extra time for porous hair

224

Finishing and Styling Hints

SPECIAL TIPS

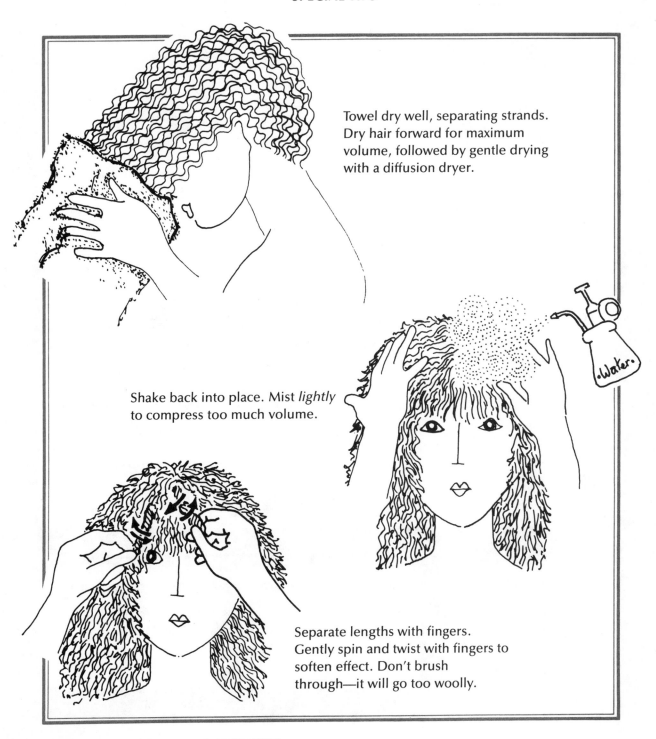

Towel dry well, separating strands. Dry hair forward for maximum volume, followed by gentle drying with a diffusion dryer.

Shake back into place. Mist *lightly* to compress too much volume.

Separate lengths with fingers. Gently spin and twist with fingers to soften effect. Don't brush through—it will go too woolly.

TOOLS AND APPLIANCES REQUIRED
Towel
Wide-tooth comb
Lamp or diffusion dryer or quartz dryer
Mist bottle
Spray shine (optional)

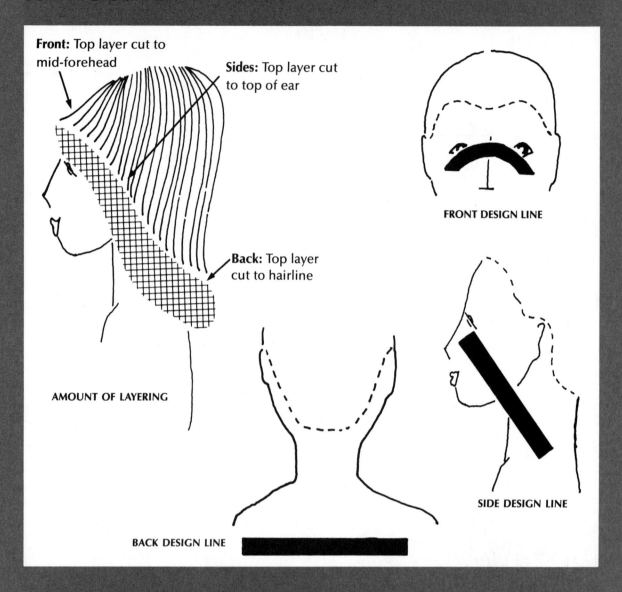

Front: Top layer cut to mid-forehead

Sides: Top layer cut to top of ear

Back: Top layer cut to hairline

AMOUNT OF LAYERING

FRONT DESIGN LINE

SIDE DESIGN LINE

BACK DESIGN LINE

THIS STYLE HIDES

Head shape
Head size
Profile
Ears
Wide face
Chin
Jawline
All hairlines
Narrow temples
Sparse hair at temples
Neck shapes: wide,
    short, long, thin

THIS STYLE HIGHLIGHTS

Thin face
Long face
Low forehead
Hair condition

BODY PROPORTIONS

Suitable for medium, tall, and large proportions

THIS IS A *MINIMUM CARE* STYLE FOR CURLY HAIR.

THIS IS A *TEMPORARY* STYLE FOR STRAIGHT HAIR.

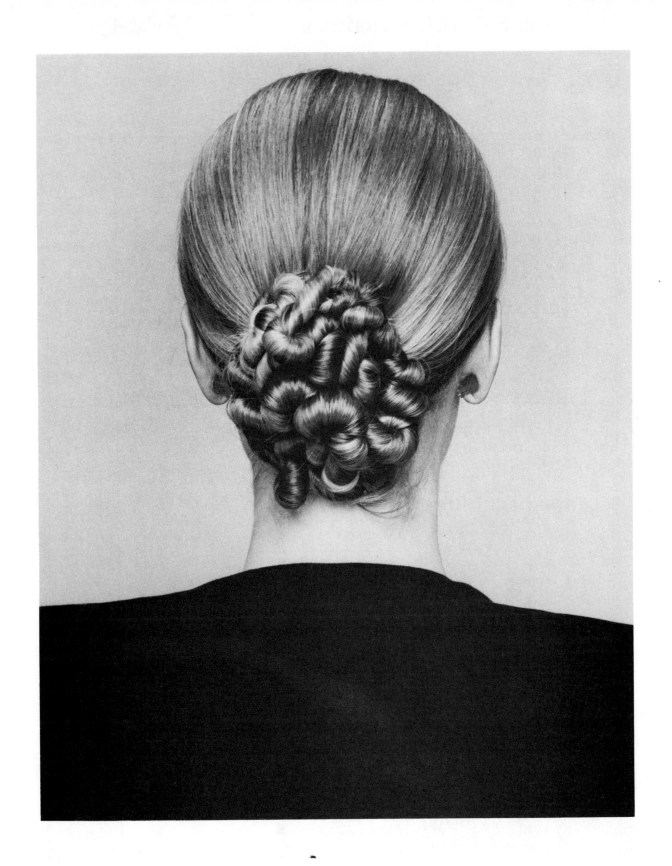

35 Uniquely neat

Your Hair's Characteristics   Stylability

TEXTURE	FORMATION	QUANTITY	HAIR TYPE	CODE	TIMING	SKILL RATING
FINE	STRAIGHT	THIN	1	■	**Note:** This style does not require freshly shampooed hair. Time estimates are for dry-hair styling.	
	STRAIGHT	MEDIUM	2	■		
	STRAIGHT	THICK	3	■		
	WAVY	THIN	4	■		
	WAVY	MEDIUM	5	■		
	WAVY	THICK	6	■		
	CURLY	THIN	7	■	20 to 30 mins.	4
	CURLY	MEDIUM	8	■		
	CURLY	THICK	9	■		
MEDIUM	STRAIGHT	THIN	10	■		
	STRAIGHT	MEDIUM	11	■		
	STRAIGHT	THICK	12	■		
	WAVY	THIN	13	■		
	WAVY	MEDIUM	14	■	20 to 30 mins.	4
	WAVY	THICK	15	■		
	CURLY	THIN	16	■		
	CURLY	MEDIUM	17	■		
	CURLY	THICK	18	■		
COARSE	STRAIGHT	THIN	19	■		
	STRAIGHT	MEDIUM	20	■		
	STRAIGHT	THICK	21	■		
	WAVY	THIN	22	■		
	WAVY	MEDIUM	23	■	20 to 30 mins.	4
	WAVY	THICK	24	■		
	CURLY	THIN	25	■		
	CURLY	MEDIUM	26	■		
	CURLY	THICK	27	■		

■ GOOD   ☐ POSSIBLE   X NOT RECOMMENDED   S STRAIGHTENING   C COLORING   WP WAVY PERM   CP CURLY PERM

Finishing and Styling Hints

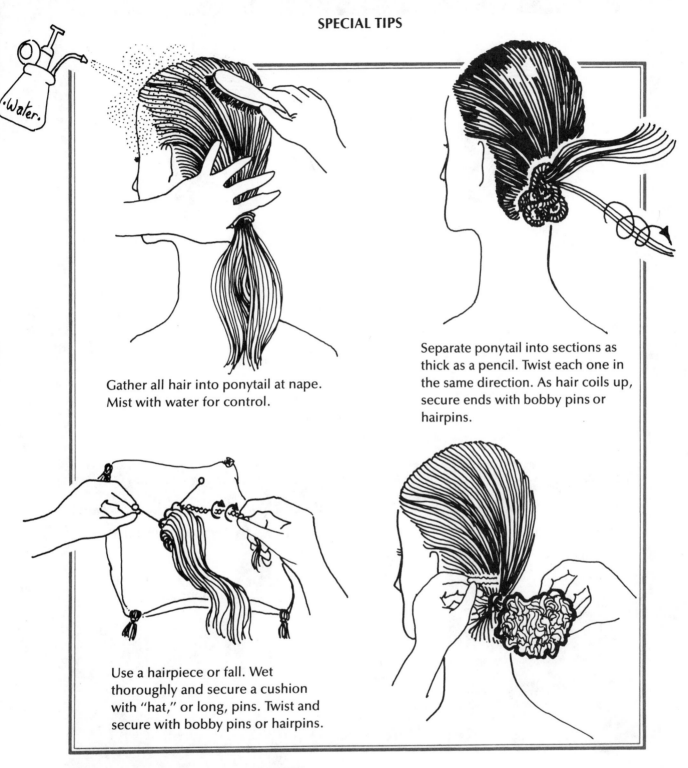

Gather all hair into ponytail at nape. Mist with water for control.

Separate ponytail into sections as thick as a pencil. Twist each one in the same direction. As hair coils up, secure ends with bobby pins or hairpins.

Use a hairpiece or fall. Wet thoroughly and secure a cushion with "hat," or long, pins. Twist and secure with bobby pins or hairpins.

TOOLS AND APPLIANCES REQUIRED

Wide-tooth comb	Bobby pins
Rattail comb	Hairpins
Flat-back brush	Covered band
Mist bottle	Gel setting lotion (optional)
Long clips	Hairpiece or fall (optional)

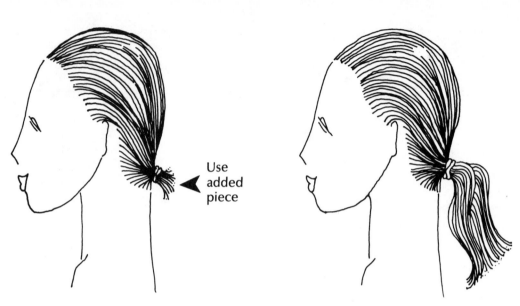

MINIMUM LENGTH REQUIRED

Long enough to gather into a ponytail at nape. The shorter the hair, the higher the tail.

Or, if the tail reaches your shoulder when gathered, the thicker your hair, the bigger the "serpents"; the thinner your hair, the smaller the "serpents."

THIS STYLE HIDES

Hair condition
Bad haircut

THIS STYLE HIGHLIGHTS

Head shape
Head size
Ears
Face shape
Chin
Jawline
All hairlines
Neck shapes: wide,
    short, long, thin

BODY PROPORTIONS

Suitable for petite, small, and medium proportions

THIS IS A *TEMPORARY* STYLE FOR ALL FORMATIONS BUT *MINIMUM CARE* WHEN STYLED INTO PLACE.

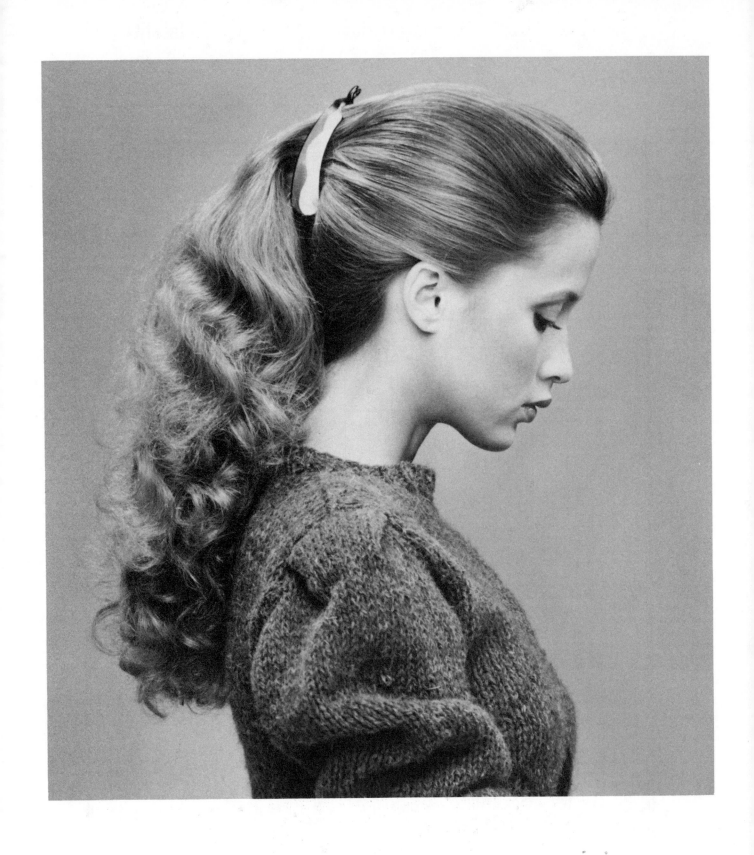

36 The brushed, gathered look for all occasions

Your Hair's Characteristics | Stylability

TEXTURE	FORMATION	QUANTITY	HAIR TYPE	CODE	TIMING*	SKILL RATING
FINE	STRAIGHT	THIN	1	WP4 ■	30 to 40 mins.; if setting only, 15 to 20 mins.	3 to 4
	STRAIGHT	MEDIUM	2	WP5 ■		
	STRAIGHT	THICK	3	WP6 ■		
	WAVY	THIN	4	C13 ■		
	WAVY	MEDIUM	5	■		
	WAVY	THICK	6	■		
	CURLY	THIN	7	C16 ☐		
	CURLY	MEDIUM	8	☐		
	CURLY	THICK	9	☐		
MEDIUM	STRAIGHT	THIN	10	WP13 ■	35 to 40 mins.; if setting only, 15 to 20 mins.	3 to 4
	STRAIGHT	MEDIUM	11	WP14 ■		
	STRAIGHT	THICK	12	WP15 ■		
	WAVY	THIN	13	C22 ■		
	WAVY	MEDIUM	14	■		
	WAVY	THICK	15	■		
	CURLY	THIN	16	C25 ☐		
	CURLY	MEDIUM	17	☐		
	CURLY	THICK	18	☐		
COARSE	STRAIGHT	THIN	19	WP22 ■	40 to 50 mins.; if setting only, 15 to 25 mins.	3 to 4
	STRAIGHT	MEDIUM	20	WP23 ■		
	STRAIGHT	THICK	21	WP24 ■		
	WAVY	THIN	22	C23 ■		
	WAVY	MEDIUM	23	■		
	WAVY	THICK	24	■		
	CURLY	THIN	25	C26 ☐		
	CURLY	MEDIUM	26	☐		
	CURLY	THICK	27	☐		

232

■ GOOD   ☐ POSSIBLE   X NOT RECOMMENDED   S STRAIGHTENING   C COLORING   WP WAVY PERM   CP CURLY PERM

*25% extra time for porous hair

Finishing and Styling Hints

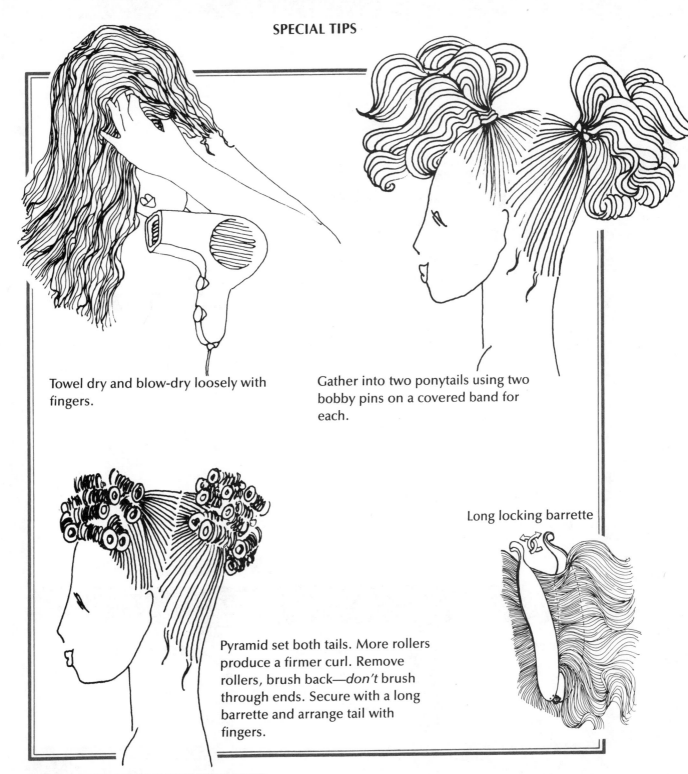

Towel dry and blow-dry loosely with fingers.

Gather into two ponytails using two bobby pins on a covered band for each.

Long locking barrette

Pyramid set both tails. More rollers produce a firmer curl. Remove rollers, brush back—*don't* brush through ends. Secure with a long barrette and arrange tail with fingers.

TOOLS AND APPLIANCES REQUIRED

Towel

Long barrette

Wide-tooth comb

Rattail comb

Flat-back brush

Blow-dryer

Hot rollers

Covered bands with bobby pins

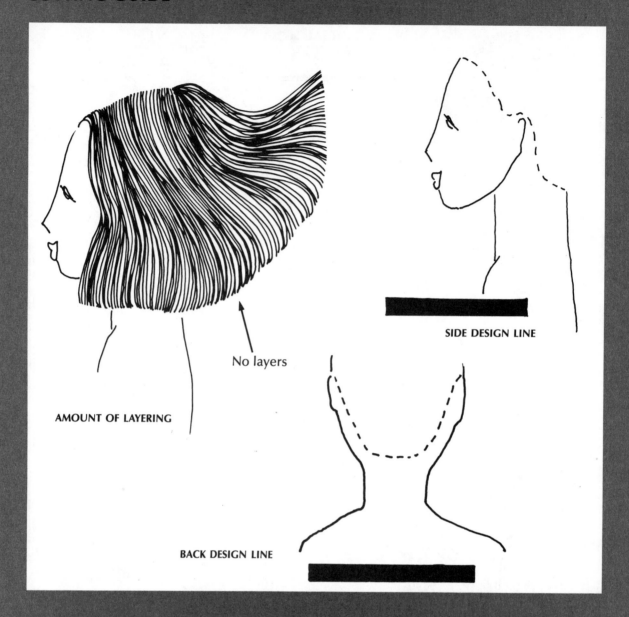

No layers

AMOUNT OF LAYERING

SIDE DESIGN LINE

BACK DESIGN LINE

THIS STYLE HIDES

Head shape
Profile
Neck shapes: wide,
  short, long, thin

THIS STYLE HIGHLIGHTS

Head size
Ears
Face shape
Chin
Jawline
All hairlines
Hair condition

BODY PROPORTIONS

Suitable for petite,
small, medium,
and tall proportions

THIS IS A *MINIMUM CARE* STYLE FOR WAVY AND CURLY HAIR.

THIS IS A *TEMPORARY* STYLE FOR STRAIGHT HAIR.

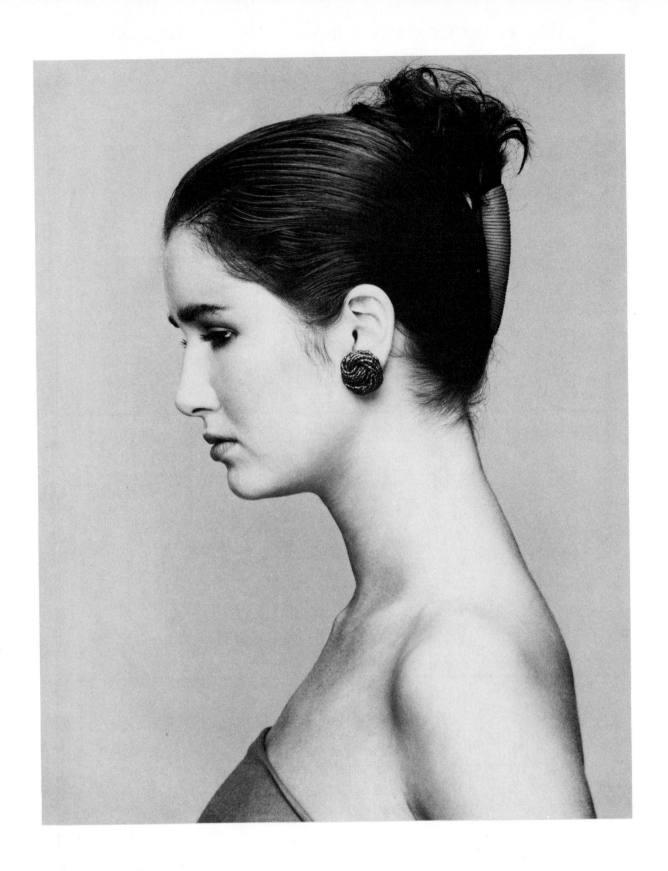

37 Bound to be beautiful

Your Hair's Characteristics | Stylability

TEXTURE	FORMATION	QUANTITY	HAIR TYPE	CODE	TIMING	SKILL RATING
FINE	STRAIGHT	THIN	1	X	**Note:** This style does not require freshly shampooed hair. Time estimates are for dry-hair styling. 10 to 20 mins.	3
FINE	STRAIGHT	MEDIUM	2	■		
FINE	STRAIGHT	THICK	3	■		
FINE	WAVY	THIN	4	X		
FINE	WAVY	MEDIUM	5	■		
FINE	WAVY	THICK	6	■		
FINE	CURLY	THIN	7	X		
FINE	CURLY	MEDIUM	8	■		
FINE	CURLY	THICK	9	■		
MEDIUM	STRAIGHT	THIN	10	X	10 to 20 mins.	3
MEDIUM	STRAIGHT	MEDIUM	11	■		
MEDIUM	STRAIGHT	THICK	12	■		
MEDIUM	WAVY	THIN	13	X		
MEDIUM	WAVY	MEDIUM	14	■		
MEDIUM	WAVY	THICK	15	■		
MEDIUM	CURLY	THIN	16	X		
MEDIUM	CURLY	MEDIUM	17	■		
MEDIUM	CURLY	THICK	18	■		
COARSE	STRAIGHT	THIN	19	X	10 to 20 mins.	3
COARSE	STRAIGHT	MEDIUM	20	■		
COARSE	STRAIGHT	THICK	21	■		
COARSE	WAVY	THIN	22	X		
COARSE	WAVY	MEDIUM	23	■		
COARSE	WAVY	THICK	24	■		
COARSE	CURLY	THIN	25	X		
COARSE	CURLY	MEDIUM	26	■		
COARSE	CURLY	THICK	27	■		

■ GOOD   □ POSSIBLE   X NOT RECOMMENDED   **S** STRAIGHTENING   **C** COLORING   **WP** WAVY PERM   **CP** CURLY PERM

SPECIAL TIPS

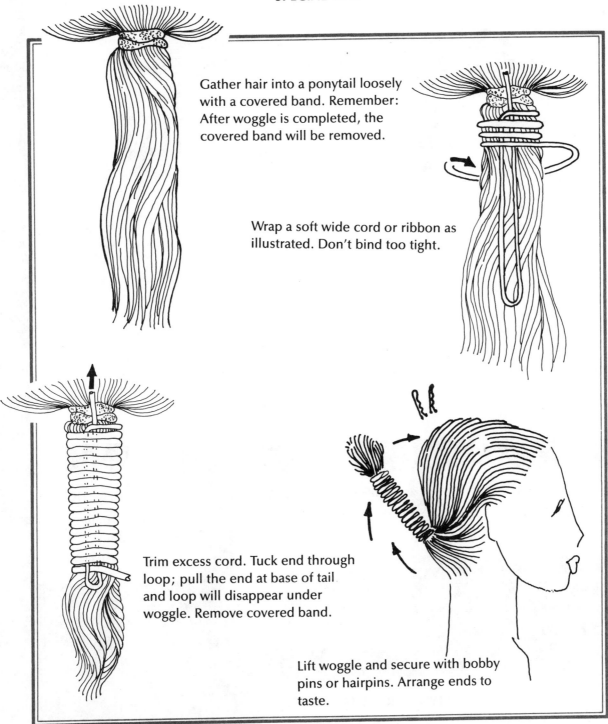

Gather hair into a ponytail loosely with a covered band. Remember: After woggle is completed, the covered band will be removed.

Wrap a soft wide cord or ribbon as illustrated. Don't bind too tight.

Trim excess cord. Tuck end through loop; pull the end at base of tail and loop will disappear under woggle. Remove covered band.

Lift woggle and secure with bobby pins or hairpins. Arrange ends to taste.

TOOLS AND APPLIANCES REQUIRED

Yard of cord or ribbon
Flat-back brush
Covered band (or covered band with bobby pins)
Mist bottle
Bobby pins or hairpins

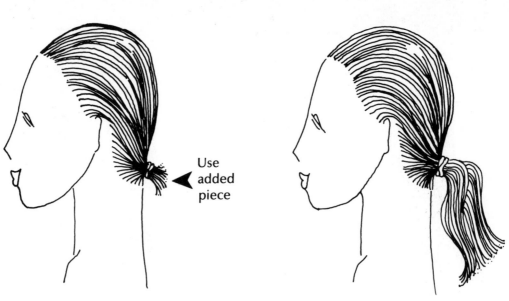

MINIMUM LENGTH REQUIRED

Long enough to gather into a ponytail at nape. The shorter the hair, the higher the tail.

Or, if the tail reaches your shoulder when gathered, the thicker your hair, the bigger the woggle; the thinner your hair, the smaller the woggle.

THIS STYLE HIDES

Hair condition
Bad haircut

THIS STYLE HIGHLIGHTS

Head shape
Face shape
Chin
Jawline
All hairlines
Neck shapes: wide,
    short, long, thin

BODY PROPORTIONS

Suitable for petite, small, medium, and tall proportions

THIS IS A *TEMPORARY* STYLE FOR ALL FORMATIONS BUT *MINIMUM CARE* WHEN STYLED INTO PLACE.

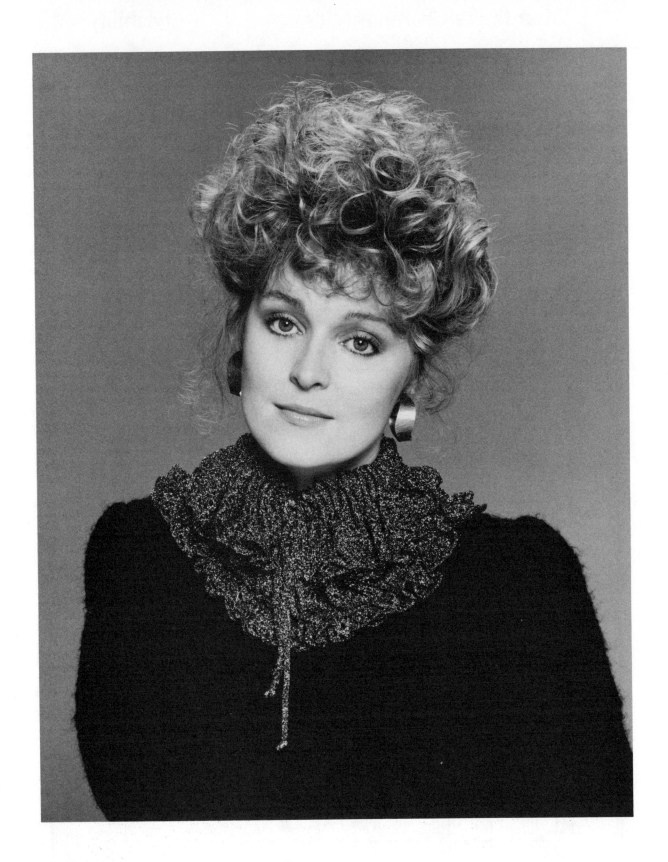

38

Pure and simple

Your Hair's Characteristics | Stylability

TEXTURE	FORMATION	QUANTITY	HAIR TYPE	CODE	TIMING	SKILL RATING
FINE	STRAIGHT	THIN	1	■	**Note:** This style does not require freshly shampooed hair. Time estimates are for dry-hair styling.	3 to 4
FINE	STRAIGHT	MEDIUM	2	■		
FINE	STRAIGHT	THICK	3	■		
FINE	WAVY	THIN	4	■		
FINE	WAVY	MEDIUM	5	■		
FINE	WAVY	THICK	6	■		
FINE	CURLY	THIN	7	■	10 to 20 mins.	
FINE	CURLY	MEDIUM	8	■		
FINE	CURLY	THICK	9	■		
MEDIUM	STRAIGHT	THIN	10	■		3 to 4
MEDIUM	STRAIGHT	MEDIUM	11	■		
MEDIUM	STRAIGHT	THICK	12	■		
MEDIUM	WAVY	THIN	13	■		
MEDIUM	WAVY	MEDIUM	14	■	10 to 20 mins.	
MEDIUM	WAVY	THICK	15	■		
MEDIUM	CURLY	THIN	16	■		
MEDIUM	CURLY	MEDIUM	17	■		
MEDIUM	CURLY	THICK	18	■		
COARSE	STRAIGHT	THIN	19	■		3 to 4
COARSE	STRAIGHT	MEDIUM	20	■		
COARSE	STRAIGHT	THICK	21	■		
COARSE	WAVY	THIN	22	■		
COARSE	WAVY	MEDIUM	23	■	10 to 20 mins.	
COARSE	WAVY	THICK	24	■		
COARSE	CURLY	THIN	25	■		
COARSE	CURLY	MEDIUM	26	■		
COARSE	CURLY	THICK	27	■		

■ GOOD   □ POSSIBLE   X NOT RECOMMENDED   **S** STRAIGHTENING   **C** COLORING   **WP** WAVY PERM   **CP** CURLY PERM

SPECIAL TIPS

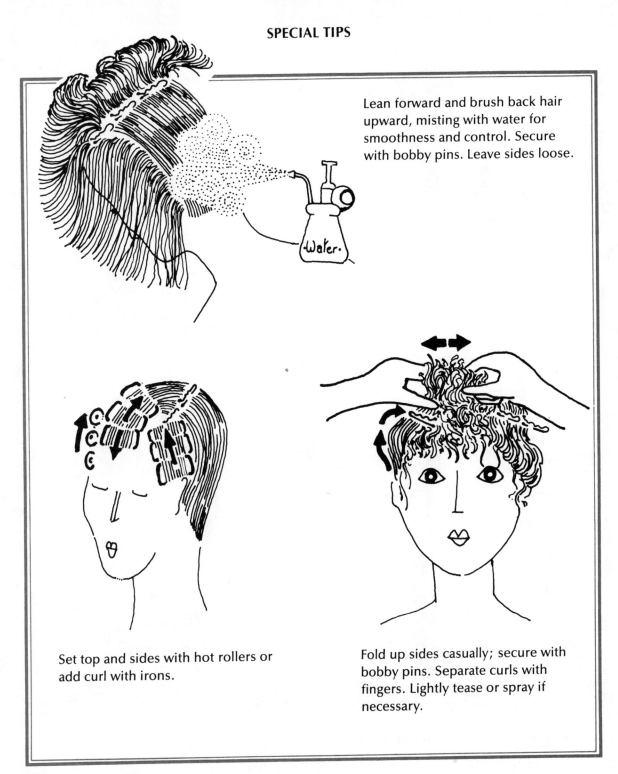

Lean forward and brush back hair upward, misting with water for smoothness and control. Secure with bobby pins. Leave sides loose.

Set top and sides with hot rollers or add curl with irons.

Fold up sides casually; secure with bobby pins. Separate curls with fingers. Lightly tease or spray if necessary.

TOOLS AND APPLIANCES REQUIRED

Rattail comb
Small-diameter curling iron or hot rollers
Mist bottle
Bobby pins
Hairpins
Flat-back brush
Hair spray (optional)

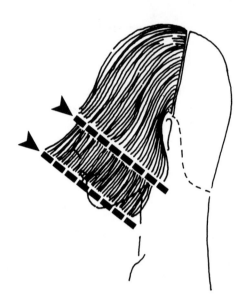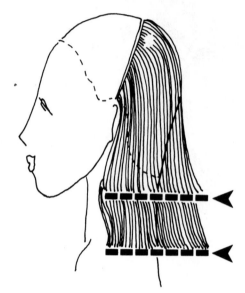

MINIMUM LENGTHS REQUIRED

Front: Top layer at least over brow.
Bottom length at least below nose.

Back: Top layer at least over hairline.
Botton length at least to shoulder.

THIS STYLE HIDES

Head shape
Head size
Receding hairline
Low forehead
Narrow temples
Sparse hair at temples
Wide temples
Front hairline
Hair condition

THIS STYLE HIGHLIGHTS

Profile
Ears
Face shape
Chin
Jawline
Nape hairline
Hairline in front of ears
Neck shapes: wide,
    short, long, thin

BODY PROPORTIONS

Suitable for petite,
small, medium,
and tall proportions

THIS IS A *TEMPORARY* STYLE FOR ALL FORMATIONS

BUT *MINIMUM CARE* FOR WAVY-TO-CURLY HAIR WHEN STYLED INTO PLACE.

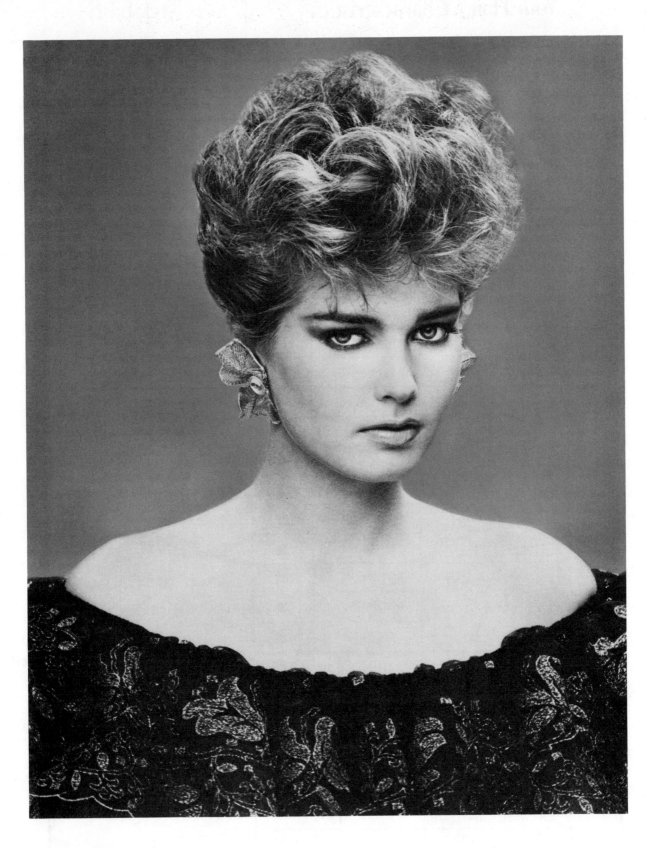

39 Short, thick, and wavy for evening

Your Hair's Characteristics | Stylability

TEXTURE	FORMATION	QUANTITY	HAIR TYPE	CODE	TIMING*	SKILL RATING
FINE	STRAIGHT	THIN	1	WP4 ■	25 to 35 mins.	3 to 4
	STRAIGHT	MEDIUM	2	WP5 ■		
	STRAIGHT	THICK	3	WP6 ■		
	WAVY	THIN	4	C13 ■		
	WAVY	MEDIUM	5	C14 ■		
	WAVY	THICK	6	■		
	CURLY	THIN	7	C16 □		
	CURLY	MEDIUM	8	□		
	CURLY	THICK	9	□		
MEDIUM	STRAIGHT	THIN	10	WP13 ■	25 to 35 mins.	3 to 4
	STRAIGHT	MEDIUM	11	WP14 ■		
	STRAIGHT	THICK	12	WP15 ■		
	WAVY	THIN	13	C22 ■		
	WAVY	MEDIUM	14	■		
	WAVY	THICK	15	■		
	CURLY	THIN	16	C25 □		
	CURLY	MEDIUM	17	■		
	CURLY	THICK	18	■		
COARSE	STRAIGHT	THIN	19	WP22 ■	30 to 40 mins.	3 to 4
	STRAIGHT	MEDIUM	20	WP23 ■		
	STRAIGHT	THICK	21	WP24 ■		
	WAVY	THIN	22	C23 ■		
	WAVY	MEDIUM	23	■		
	WAVY	THICK	24	■		
	CURLY	THIN	25	C26 □		
	CURLY	MEDIUM	26	□		
	CURLY	THICK	27	□		

■ GOOD   □ POSSIBLE   X NOT RECOMMENDED   S STRAIGHTENING   C COLORING   WP WAVY PERM   CP CURLY PERM

244

*25% extra time for porous hair

Finishing and Styling Hints

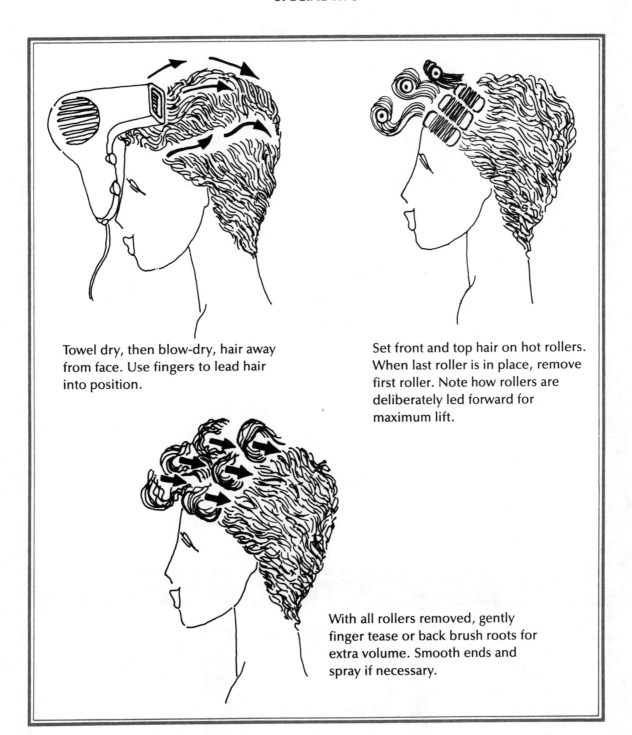

Towel dry, then blow-dry, hair away from face. Use fingers to lead hair into position.

Set front and top hair on hot rollers. When last roller is in place, remove first roller. Note how rollers are deliberately led forward for maximum lift.

With all rollers removed, gently finger tease or back brush roots for extra volume. Smooth ends and spray if necessary.

TOOLS AND APPLIANCES REQUIRED

Towel
Wide-tooth comb
Rattail comb
Blow-dryer
Hot rollers
Hair spray (optional)

CUTTING GUIDE

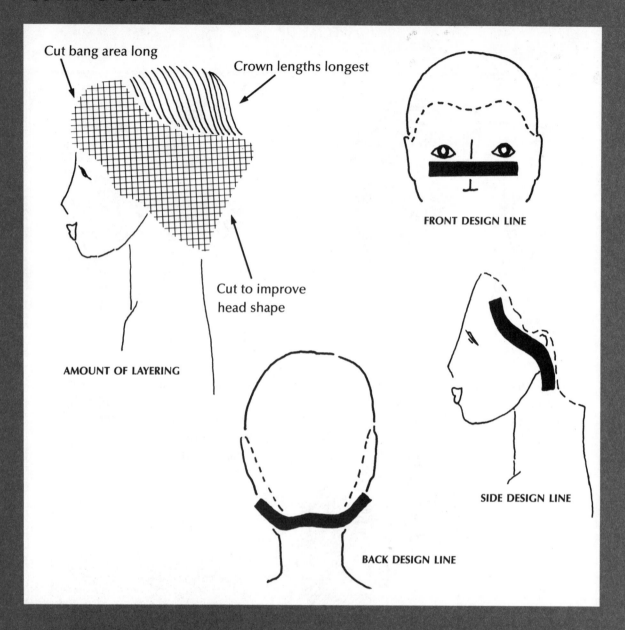

Cut bang area long

Crown lengths longest

Cut to improve head shape

AMOUNT OF LAYERING

FRONT DESIGN LINE

SIDE DESIGN LINE

BACK DESIGN LINE

THIS STYLE HIDES

Head shape
Hair condition
Low nape hairline
Low forehead

THIS STYLE HIGHLIGHTS

Short face
Chin
Jawline
Hairline in front of ears

BODY PROPORTIONS
Suitable for medium-to-tall proportions

THIS IS A *TEMPORARY* STYLE FOR ALL FORMATIONS.

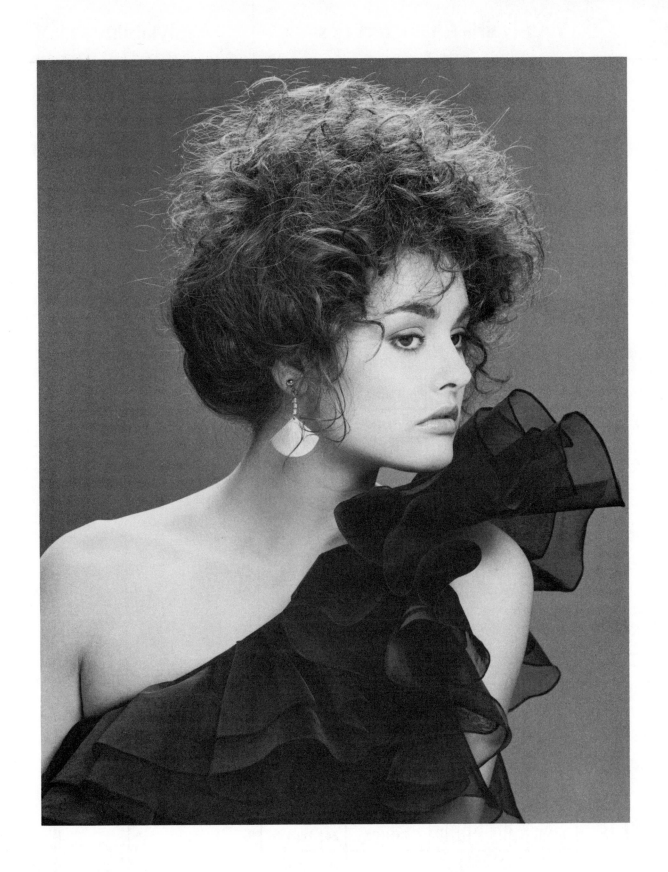

40 Foxy lady

Your Hair's Characteristics

Stylability

TEXTURE	FORMATION	QUANTITY	HAIR TYPE	CODE	TIMING	SKILL RATING
FINE	STRAIGHT	THIN	1	X	**Note:** This style does not require freshly shampooed hair. Time estimates are for dry-hair styling. 10 to 20 mins.	3 to 4
FINE	STRAIGHT	MEDIUM	2	X		
FINE	STRAIGHT	THICK	3	X		
FINE	WAVY	THIN	4	C13 ☐		
FINE	WAVY	MEDIUM	5	☐		
FINE	WAVY	THICK	6	☐		
FINE	CURLY	THIN	7	C16 ■		
FINE	CURLY	MEDIUM	8	■		
FINE	CURLY	THICK	9	■		
MEDIUM	STRAIGHT	THIN	10	CP16 ■	10 to 20 mins.	3 to 4
MEDIUM	STRAIGHT	MEDIUM	11	CP17 ■		
MEDIUM	STRAIGHT	THICK	12	CP18 ■		
MEDIUM	WAVY	THIN	13	C22 ☐		
MEDIUM	WAVY	MEDIUM	14	☐		
MEDIUM	WAVY	THICK	15	☐		
MEDIUM	CURLY	THIN	16	C25 ■		
MEDIUM	CURLY	MEDIUM	17	■		
MEDIUM	CURLY	THICK	18	■		
COARSE	STRAIGHT	THIN	19	X	10 to 20 mins.	3 to 4
COARSE	STRAIGHT	MEDIUM	20	X		
COARSE	STRAIGHT	THICK	21	X		
COARSE	WAVY	THIN	22	C23 ☐		
COARSE	WAVY	MEDIUM	23	☐		
COARSE	WAVY	THICK	24	☐		
COARSE	CURLY	THIN	25	C26 ■		
COARSE	CURLY	MEDIUM	26	■		
COARSE	CURLY	THICK	27	■		

■ GOOD   ☐ POSSIBLE   X NOT RECOMMENDED   S STRAIGHTENING   C COLORING   WP WAVY PERM   CP CURLY PERM

Finishing and Styling Hints

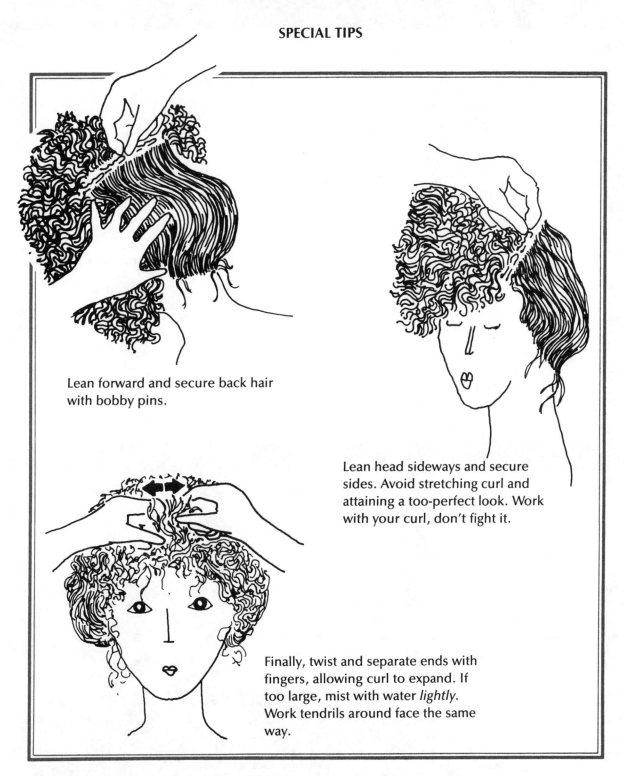

Lean forward and secure back hair with bobby pins.

Lean head sideways and secure sides. Avoid stretching curl and attaining a too-perfect look. Work with your curl, don't fight it.

Finally, twist and separate ends with fingers, allowing curl to expand. If too large, mist with water *lightly*. Work tendrils around face the same way.

TOOLS AND APPLIANCES REQUIRED

Wide-tooth comb
Rattail comb
Bobby pins
Hairpins
Flat-back brush
Spray shine (optional)
Hair spray (optional)

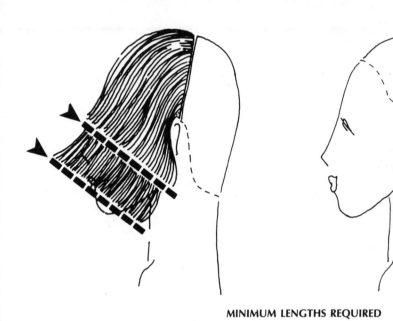

MINIMUM LENGTHS REQUIRED

Front: Top layers at least over brow. Bottom lengths at least below nose.

Back: Top layer at least over hairline. Bottom length at least to shoulder.

THIS STYLE HIDES

Head shape
Head size
Profile
Ears
Wide face
Receding hairline
Low forehead
Narrow temples
Sparse hair at temples
Wide temples
Front hairline
Hairline in front of ears
Hair condition
Bad haircut

THIS STYLE HIGHLIGHTS

Thin face
Short face
Long face
Chubby cheeks
Chin
Jawline
Nape hairline
Neck shapes: wide,
    short, long, thin

BODY PROPORTIONS

Suitable for medium, tall, and large proportions

THIS IS A *MINIMUM CARE* STYLE FOR CURLY HAIR.

THIS IS A *TEMPORARY* STYLE FOR WAVY AND STRAIGHT HAIR.